BECOMING

NURSE AWESOME

LOVE NOTES
+
LIFE LESSONS

FOR THE BRAND NEW NURSE

This book is dedicated to life and to

My parents who gave it
My son who saved it
My husband who completes it
My friends who support it
My family who enrich it
My fellow nurses who share it

My patients who bless it

CHAPTER LISTING

In the Beginning...I used the phrase, 'Way to Go Nurse Awesome' to lovingly describe the not-always-stellar-but-always-heart-felt clinical abilities of both myself and my classmates during our 1st semester of nursing school. We were mostly all thumbs but we were also all-heart in action!

Then, as time passed + school got super-tough, I'd use the label 'Nurse Awesome' to bolster the spirits of me and my peers as we all wondered whether we had what it took to even finish school.

Finally, it evolved to be a tiny mantra of encouragement when one of those particularly sticky days that nursing invariably brings would jump up to surprise me.

As I began making videos and helping other nurses develop their study chops it felt natural to keep using the phrase ***Nurse Awesome*** to address 'my people'.

Throughout this book when you these words think of them as:

> A point of encouragement for tough days

> A reminder of your own badassery

> A tool in your ninja pack; to be used when awesome is the only medicine that will fix the crazy

> A foundational belief on which to build your new practice

Nurse Awesome is a noun + a verb. It describes your heart, your spirit and the superhero work you get to do as a registered nurse.

Thanks for dedicating your life to helping other people make their own life a better place to be. In case you ever doubt it let me remind you how brilliantly your light shines. You are such a blessing to this world.

INTRODUCTION

My name is Melissa + I am so happy to meet you!

Welcome to the registered nurse club. Otherwise known as the only job in the world where you get to experience the highs and lows of human existence daily. We endure some fierce + frustrating initiation rituals before we are ready to use our new ninja-skills and let the world call us 'their nurse', huh?

I dig the patients that I care for each shift and empowering them is one of the big 'whys' behind my practice. I love that sharing my time + heart can help them improve their lives. It is a pretty cool way to earn a living and make a positive impact on the world. Despite being blessed by those souls that are the reason for my job, it is you, my fellow nursing phenoms that get my full attention in these pages. Patients can wait for another day.

After all, you've just spent the better part of every waking second over the last few years learning the science behind this career; you deserve some TLC now. I know a lot of that time has been in a skills lab somewhere inserting this or that into dummies that can't move or cry or curse at you. Even so, this book is not about the hard skills you need as a new nurse. You've no doubt got those skills on lock!

This book, well, it is about the soft stuff. The sticky stuff no one really teaches in school; the stuff that is hard to define but that we spend a ton of time dealing with on the daily anyway. We are going to talk about the art of nursing here. That stuff behind all the hard skills of your practice.

Yea, I said it. Nursing is both a science and an art. Heavy, right? As much as the left-brained logical among us might like to think there is only room for science here, you just can't function in this world without your heart. Likewise, you will get nowhere fast if you rely strictly on your heart and leave the science piece out.

You need both to be an awesome nurse.

I was elated when I graduated nursing school and downright joyful when I passed my NCLEX exam. While I had adjusted to the intensity and idiosyncrasies of school I somehow believed that my first actual nursing job would be a blissful reward for all my efforts. Not so much. I left many shifts wondering out loud to the sky, 'Is THIS what nursing is really all about?' Even more days I left pleading,

'Puh-lease, do not let THIS be what nursing is all about!'

I questioned why I had ventured from my cushy corporate gig into the land of crazy. I felt in the core of my being that me + nursing was one huge-ass mistake.

Let me be clear. While you've worked hard to gain your new skill set, you are about to work even harder to figure out how to use those new skills 'in the real world' without losing your shit in the process.

This first year, as you learn to think like a nurse, I swear you will catch yourself reflecting back on those crazy NCLEX questions and wondering why you thought they were so hard. You will wish for the safety of the school you couldn't wait to get away from and you will question yourself; a lot.

The real-world NCLEX questions that play out in front of you thru each shift will be more than a little hard and plenty of those situations will make you feel small and stupid. You will feel scared in a way that you never have to this point.

Something about life and death does that to a person.

Don't sweat this though, sweet pea. There will be plenty of stuff that does NOT suck. Lots of days come along where you will feel like you actually deserve the license they gave you and many times you will think, 'Holy cow! I am smarter than I thought. I am actually an awesome nurse!'

Consider this to be a trail of breadcrumbs to help you find that place a little faster. I created it because I don't want anyone that comes after me to have to spend time feeling so small and incapable. Truth is, you are powerful beyond measure. Besides, you have way too much goodness to share with the world to be letting fear wonk up your time.

It is not a scholarly text. It is a love note about the lessons I've learned set down like a chat between friends. You should know that I write like I speak (much to the dismay of my former editors), I am a Texan and there is plenty a colorful phrase thrown about in these pages. Despite that, you outta learn some useful stuff to help ya navigate thru these first months as a nurse.

I believe you will leave feeling as if you have a solid grasp on a whole lot of the stuff you didn't know you needed to know, a better understanding of the stuff you already know you don't know, and an action plan to ferret out the stuff that threatens to suck the joy out of your practice; and all the bits in between.

You already know that your prime directive this first year as a nurse is to create a rock solid practice based on the foundations you laid down in school.

Do you also know that this time is also about finding your focus as a nurse while having some fun with those rescue ninja skills that you worked your butt off to learn? Indeed this will be the bulk of your work as you come out of the gates into nursing proper.

It is about finding your own special medicine and how to give it to your patients. It is about learning who you are as a nurse, learning your boundaries and learning to love the world in a way that only you can love.

Mostly, it is time for you to learn the importance of nurturing yourself; not just your patients.

And here you thought learning to prioritize was your main objective. Sure, there is that but it is just a small, small piece of all the goodness in store for you this year.

It might not feel like it much this first year in your new gig but you and I are blessed to get to do this work.

This nursing gig is sacred work and right this second, even as a new nurse; every action you take carries with it the power to heal.

Yes, you. You are a healer.

Your full presence has the power to transform every single person it encounters. If I have my way, by the end of this book you will know that to be truer than any other thing you have spent the last few years learning at school.

You, my new friend, are both a life-saver + a life-changer.

You already ARE Nurse Awesome so don't let anything that happens in this first year convince you otherwise.

Let's get to it...

"I've learned that people will forget what you said, people will forget what you did, but people will never forget how you made them feel."

Maya Angelou

Dear 1st week of my new job—

No matter how many times you try to convince me that I learned nothing in school + that I suck…

I don't believe it.

I will not waste my energy on fear but instead keep my head down and focused on absorbing everything I can right now. I will not believe you when you make me feel stupid; I am not stupid..I am awesome!

I will quickly regroup when I feel overwhelmed. I will rest when needed and ask for floaties when drowning! I have everything in me that I need to be an awesome nurse

I am in a safe place, my school taught me

well. I've got this on lock...

So bring on all ya got—Me

ENTER FEAR, STAGE RIGHT

The last few months of nursing school go by in a flash, huh?

Years of dreaming about being a nurse, entrance exams, volunteer work, job-hunting, school cliques and the semesters of never-ending care plans are all behind you.

You are done becoming a nurse, time to be one!

Stop here. Savor this spot. This feeling of elation, the happy dance you can't stop doing, the smile that will not leave your face, the pride you feel for having done this something that threatened every step of each semester to be something you could not do.

Well deserved, all of it. Way to go, Nurse Awesome!

When I finally arrived at this spot the only thing I could think was, 'Holy shit, I am finally a nurse, now what?'

I mean really, every ounce of everything in my life at that point was consumed by nursing school. Now that it was time to actually nurse, I was not sure what was next.

You might experience this same feeling. It is an odd mix of elation and excitement with a touch of uncertainty thrown in. Don't let it steal your joy here.

There were plenty of times in school when I thought I was just never going to make it out. In spite of it, I had actually jumped all the hurdles school put in front of me. I was proud and ready to be an awesome nurse that contributed positive to the lives of all my patients.

Floating on that cloud of 'holycrapiamdone-ness', well, the last thing I was feeling in this moment was fear.

At least that is what I thought...

> We had just taken our last nursing school exam ever. A bunch of us were in the atrium waiting for our respective buddies to be done with their exam so the celebratory margaritas could commence. We chatted excitedly about the fact that we were finally done with school. There is a crazy high your get walking out of theory class for the last time that your non-nurse friends will never understand.
>
> Then right in the middle of that high came this little voice with a question for all of us that none of us expected.
>
> 'Aren't any of y'all scared?'

I was thrown a little by the 'pause' from stage right:

Uhm, no, I have been preparing for this day for years. Are you kidding me? Afraid? Me? I am the girl of steel. I have confidence for days. There is not any way at all that I am feeling afraid.

Until I did. There it was an uneasy feeling in my gut. Smack in the middle of my classmates simple question, mixed in with all the celebrations of 'done-ness' and happiness at being ready to start my new career.

My classmates' courage to speak out about what some of us felt allowed an admission that 'yes, within our joy we were all a bit freaked out about leaving school and being on our own.'

This got the whole lot of us talking. She was most concerned about the NCLEX. Other peers were freaked that the safety net of instructors in the middle of a crisis would be removed or that they would forget everything learned. Still others were just afraid they would find out they were not cut-out for the world we were entering and they would be a crappy nurse. Others simply worried about finding jobs at all in our saturated marketplace.

What are you feeling afraid about right now, as you move away from school? It is totally normal to have some butterflies mixed in among the happy, so don't sweat it if you feel some here..

Me? Well, I was nervous about jumping from protection of professors straight into an ICU. While everyone else had started studying for the NCLEX I was hard at the critical care books, learning as much as I could about the world I was entering soon. I am a good tester so NCLEX was a little blip on the radar for me and not anything I was worried about passing.

As I walked to my car that day, the last day I would be at that campus, in that classroom, with those people; ever, I was worried that somehow, someway, after everything I had put myself and my family through to become a nurse that I would actually be a crappy nurse.

That I would kill a patient because of some bit of info I missed in the newness of my newness. That I had made a huge mistake leaving the confines of the corporate world and that I had glamorized nursing so much that I would ultimately be disappointed. I was afraid I would fail. Simple.

By the time I buckled myself into the car after that last exam

I was in full-on panic about the degree to which I would surely suck as a nurse.

Jitters are normal. A little bit of fear keeps you alert which keeps you growing and evolving as nurse. It helps you avoid complacency and can help keep your ego in check.

All good qualities to have when you are interested in keeping people alive, right? But me, I let those simple jitters morph into some big monster of doubt in the days that followed. I questioned everything about myself and what I knew as a fledgling nurse. Overachiever that I am, it did not take me long to realize I did not know much and that was going to be a huge problem.

I had really never considered this place before now. I was scared; not nervous or jittery. I was freaked out. I had zero clue how to process this much freakin fear, let alone move through it.

I consider myself a mature adult. I have been through crisis before, hell I used to manage crisis for a living. I was a single mom for 9 years so I have felt some damn stress in my life. This should not be the issue it was becoming for me.

Why then was there this sudden surge of panic that I could not control? I think it was a deep-in-my-bones knowing that it was now my ship to steer or sink that made me wanna crawl up in a corner and stay there. Forever.

Yep, no more help from the preceptor. No more instructors to ask before I took action. No more wicked-smart nurse buddies to bounce my care plans off of before I actually did the care.

To be clear, by steer or sink I mean succeed or fail, and, by ship I mean my entire darn nursing career. And, by nursing career I mean the one where people live or die because of the choices I make each shift.

Ding, Ding, Ding, there was the REAL fear factor. Life or death and me having some part in that for someone other than me. Gawd, that was my totally my freak-out factor.

I remember of particular concern was the whole ICU thing. I 'felt' prepared but in that day after theory class I was bombarded with people telling me how scared I 'outta' be and how 'crazy' I was for starting in such an intense place. (**Note to Self:** Don't listen to doubters)

A few of my classmates told me how they just couldn't imagine me in that kind of environment because I was too 'right-brained' for the logic required to be successful in the unit. I even heard flat out that I 'would be sorry' I didn't take an easier gig right out of school in order to give myself time to transition from school to practice.
I know they meant well. Most of those people were happy for me and were just expressing their own fears but damn, I took them on as my own fear and I started digging a helluva hole to escape. The next few weeks for me?

Well... I had many conversations with my husband and nursing buddy about going into Hospice instead of Intensive Care. Innumerable chats in my head about why I needed to NOT be an ICU nurse. I still remember the look on my friends face after having spent the last 2 years talking about an ICU gig. It was wholly confused and pretty priceless.

I interviewed for several Hospice jobs. I got some offers that I almost took simply because I was listening to my fear.

The big fear, that I would kill someone, was removed if people were already in Hospice care, right? I know that makes me seem like a horrible person. It was the predominant thought in my head in those moments though: if I F-up and kill someone it doesn't matter.

Point is that I let my classmate's simple question spin me into a sea of fear. I let another person's assessment of the situation guide my choices and dictate my feelings. The others felt afraid; I was supposed to as well, right?

Wrong again. I had already learned this lesson in my non-nursing life back in the days of single motherhood. Feeling fear and allowing it to paralyze you and remove what power you do have over the situation is always choice + not needed unless you say it is needed.

On top of letting fear run the ship for a bit I was violating the first rule of nursing; ahem... Always assess things for *yourself* before you take action. Always....as in ...

Nevertakeanotherpersonswordforsomethingthatrequi resanaction

Damn, I neglected to assess things for myself first and I was a train-wreck of emotion inside because of it.

Are you feeling afraid about this first 'real' nursing gig, too?

Here is how I myself out of it.

I just let myself be afraid. Really.

And I mean I let my imagination run wild with all the havoc my craptastic nursing skills caused to my patients each shift. At least once a day I killed someone in my head by some stupid mistake I made and at least once a day I lost my license as a result of some horrific and accidental action that I took without knowing that it was going to have a bad consequence.

I let my thoughts run to the extreme cause I knew that as long as I was ignoring the thoughts they would persist.

So, I spent at least a day in the horrible what-if's, you know? What kind of craziness does your mind imagine you will cause?

Here are a few of mine:

- What if I to check patient allergies and gave them something that harmed them?
- What if I used the wrong medical term to describe something and looked like an idiot?
- What if I gave the wrong medication?
- What if I tell the doctor wrong information?
- What if I fail to see a symptom before it hurts my patient?
- What if being right-brained meant I was too stupid and caring for ICU?
- What if I forgot all my training the moment I was standing in front of a patient?
- What If I suddenly just froze at the moment my patient needed me most.
- What if I forgot how to do CPR?
- What if I killed someone? What if I lost my license?

Go on and make a list of your own now. What kind of terrifying things have you imagined about your new career?

Come on, I know you have conjured up some crazy disasters in your head. May as well just get it out of your system now and let yourself get good and petrified.

Let your imagination run to the extreme. The crazy thoughts are not going to just going to go away. You have to do something about it.

Let your mind run wild. Go on, kill someone with your negligence.

Now that you've gone to that place, let's make a plan to change it, alright?

Cause man, the negative energy swirling around the fear-stuff is not at all enjoyable and totally not needed.

My personal plan of action to overcome this sort of bull crap came about by total accident.

It was crisis management I learned in my past job with corporate peeps that helped me most. I used it to help myself when school first started and then started using it to help other nurses bridge the gap from school to practice. It is easy + it works.

Some background for reference: I went to work for a large hospital system, in an Intensive Care Unit. I left school an excited, confident and capable nurse close to the top of my class (thinking I knew a lot) and ready to immerse myself in critical care.

Smiley General had an awesome reputation and they had fashioned a new nurse orientation that was both in-depth + that covered the hospitals' interests thoroughly.

I was fully steeped in mission statements, JCAHO rules, and corporate culture but they left out a lot of stuff. The gap between student nurse and actual nurse was something that I had no clue even existed as I was going through my orientation period so I didn't know I needed to ask someone to fill in the blanks for me.

When things got rolling post-orientation I had no idea how I was going to survive let alone thrive as a 'real' nurse.

It took me 2 days on shift to figure out I knew nothing, 3 months of OJT to relax a bit and another 3 to begin to love nursing as much as I thought I would when I started the whole process some 4 years past.

The first step I took to get 'okay' with my practice(and I use okay very loosely here)was to actually look at those things I thought would be catastrophic events or my new career and reframe them in the context of reality rather than the dark expanse of my imagination.

So on one side of the paper list your fear and then directly across from write out what you think might happen that would be bad for you or your patient in the form of a 'what-if' statement. Read that 'what-if' fearish thing out loud in the first person, 'as-if' it has already happened. Either speak out loud or write down the thing that you would tell your best buddy if they had confided in you that they had this fear.

Here are some of my examples:

'What-if I use the wrong medical term to describe something and sound like dumbass?

Become: 'Holy Crap I just said tachycardic when I meant tachypneic.'

My response if a friend had shared this with me: 'Thank god everyone knows you are human now' It is highly likely that you will use the wrong medical word again in your long and awesome career shake it off, toots. No one but you is still thinking about this anyway. '

Or this...

'What if I forget if their pupils are a 2 or 3 on my assessment?'

Became: 'Holy crap I forgot, were those pupils a 2 or a 3?'

To my friend: 'Seriously cut yourself some slack, sister. You are gonna forget stuff, that's what paper and pen are for, besides you can always go into the room and check again. Remember, unless they are unequal, nonreactive, or blown wide open, 'size', is largely a judgment call that again, does not end your career, harm your patient or cause the doom in your fraidey cat head to come true.'

And even with my worst fears...

'What-if I forget how to do CPR and my patient needs it?'

Became: 'Jesus H, I forgot how to put the backboard under my patient when I started CPR, what a moron I am!'

To my friend: 'No worries, you have some amazing peers around you and they will remind you until the day you do not forget anymore'

I must have had 20 pages of fears and the supportive response by the time I was done with this exercise.

Each negative thought was considered and by the time I was done and a couple of patterns emerged.

I was being uncharacteristically dramatic. I was a lot of things but I was not a drama queen so I needed to cut that out quick. Second, I was taking every single thought to the extreme. Again, not like me and something I needed to put the kibosh on posthaste. All that unchecked fear was really making me nuts!

I know this seems like a super-simple exercise and it is one. I swear if you will value yourself enough to do it you will see a tremendous change in the attitude with which you approach your day. The whole victim/I am a new nurse/I suck thing will be gone.

When I was done I was feeling about 30 lbs lighter and re-centered in my kapow. I was also seriously laughing my butt off at my own mental shenanigans.

It also made me realize that dramatic or not, all the fear I was projecting in the future was making it hard to focus on the present; which is the only place you can truly have any affect one anyway, right? (**Note to Self**: This nursing gig is not all unicorns + rainbows nor is it all trolls and thunderstorms.)

So take some time here and let your mind run wild. Be as dramatic as you like, this is just between us.

Can you see a pattern that is not really like you? Are you projecting fear into the future of your awesome nursing career?

Here is the thing. No matter how excellent your school experience was you are going to suck + be afraid, sometimes.

You are going to be stressed out and horrible things WILL happen, sometimes. There will also be days when you don't suck and things go surprisingly well; even in the first few crazy weeks of your new practice.

Your inner-awesome will show through! Nothing will remove the intensity that comes when you are charged to care for another person's life and more specifically; when you deal with death.

Let yourself feel afraid. There is no grading now. Let yourself know that there is a lot that you simply cannot, will not, should not know at this point.

Instead of allowing those simple points of fact get to be horrific show-stopper monsterish thoughts in your noggin because you ignore them just follow this lead.
Work it out with this 3 step tool and move on.

1. Turn your fear into a what-if question.

2. Say it out loud in the first person as a statement of fact like it already happened.

3. Give yourself the advice you would give your best nursing buddy that needs some reminding of their awesome.

The space between NCLEX passed and job found can allow some negative self-talk to creep in where you don't expect.

Best bet here is just to recognize it and then let it go.

I found it easier when I used the phrase, 'It is what it is...'

Seriously, consider it a new tool in your arsenal of awesome.

Some people feel this is a phrase used when people give up. Others use it to procrastinate and keep their lives from moving forward. In this case it is neither of those things.

It is incredibly useful as a tool to redirect negative thinking and snap yourself back to reality and from spiraling into self doubt or worry when you do not have an answer you 'think' you are supposed to have as THE nurse. I used this phrase a lot in the beginning. It refocused me quickly in a find out what you can and let go of the rest kind of way. I still use it daily.

The other empowering thing I did during this time was to go back to my books and learn those things that I was unfamiliar with, no matter how simple they seemed. You've known nursing is a lifelong learning pursuit for a while so no sense in explaining this further. Just be proactive and take responsibility for your learning.

Y'all seriously, in my head, before I ever even started my job I was responsible for a ton of sentinel events. You know the kind of horrible nursing mistakes that you read about in the papers? That was me. I was pretty harsh on myself and I had not even started being a nurse yet.

Do not do this to yourself, okay?

The first few months of nursing will not be neat and tidy. They will be freaking hard. You will be exhausted.

You can totally rock the socks off the first few months in spite of the hard stuff.

So, put this book down and spend some time with your fear that is dressed up in all those 'what-if's' running around in your head. If you don't have any now then keep reading and dog-ear this page for later.

Once I navigated past my fear I got a bit more realistic. I wasn't thinking I would be Florence Nightingale anymore. I also lost the notion that I would kill patients daily. (**Note to Self**: it is all about balance).

The new middle ground in my own brain, minus the what-if bull, sounded like this:

- I was going to be learning new things daily
- I will never be perfect
- I was going to ruffle feathers at times; docs included

- I was not going to have all the answers in crisis
- I was going to pause + I was going to question myself
- I was going to ask questions + feel stupid at times
- I was going to mess up even previously mastered tasks

Good thing I figured out how to get past fear and doing stupid things before I went into my job.

I didn't have to wait long to feel totally unqualified and dumb at my new gig at Smiley General.

Case in point...

At my school, hanging IV piggyback medication was a second semester skill for us. I was confident with this task. I did not for one second question my ability to successfully hang medications via piggyback. When my preceptor turned me loose with medications by the middle of my first shift it was the boost of confidence I needed in a time I was feeling somewhat less than nurse awesome material. I was happy, ready to prove that I WAS actually a nurse that was quite awesome. Then it all imploded!

> I was not prepared for what I saw when I went into the patients room to hang a piggyback of potassium. The patient was well enough, DKA + HTN, on the lower end of acuity for ICU. Still, as a new graduate with most of my experience in med-surg units I was a bit lost when I looked at the IV setup and saw 6 chambers of IV pump in use. I wanted to run. Each was running something into a huge line of stop cocks attached to a central line in the patients' internal jugular vein. None of the lines were labeled except for at the pump. I had no idea what was going where or what was compatible with the potassium I needed to

hang. I remembered that sodium bicarbonate doesn't play nicely with most drugs and that I could not run potassium in the peripheral IV line in the patients forearm. It took me ten minutes just to decipher which med was going where then another 5 to cipher the compatibility in the computer. Finally, I got all that square, put the bicarb on the peripheral IV, hung the IVPB and was out of the room. My preceptor told me I was slow but did a great job with it. I felt good until we went back into the patient's room an hour later. My preceptor reached behind the pillow + pulled up the end of the IVPB that I had forgotten to attach to the actual primary IV before starting the pump. There was a nice puddle of med on the floor behind the patient and she just winked at me and said, 'I think we are ready for the next bag of potassium now.' I looked up to see her dangling the end of the line behind the patients' head where only the two of us could see it. Yes, it was dripping behind the bed and yes, I didn't even hook it up to the patient and yes, I felt like a moron.

There was not one bit 'good' I could find with my failure.

I was given the chance to prove myself and I sucked; big time! By the time the day above was done I was so closed a crow bar could not have opened me up. I approached everything else I did that shift from a closed and fearful space. If I could make a mistake with something so simple how on earth could I do the big things I would need to in ICU? *(Note to Self:* working under this pressure must be the reason the instructors in school put so much pressure on y'all in skills lab. I get it now... it was never because they hated us.)

This day helped me forget about my anger at school for leaving things out of their teaching. More important though, it taught me a huge amount of humility; it let me see how easy shit happens when you get overloaded with stress. It engrained in my head the importance of that middle ground I talk about above. It taught me to be careful + double check the small stuff as well as not to be cocky or over-confident.

It sucked but it was totally needed 'suck' for me.

It helped demolish that perfectionist view in my head, the thought that I should know-it-all and it helped me figure out that there was going to be a huge learning curve as a new nurse. What's more, it showed me that obsessing about any of it was not helpful for me. It did not make me suddenly more experienced. Nope, worry just left me more frazzled. I needed to choose different thoughts.
No closed up thinking or auto-pilot allowed in nursing.

Huge lesson.

The other thing I started to do pretty quickly to shore myself up against the blues was to spend some time at the end of each shift reflecting on the shift. ALL parts of it rather than just what I did wrong.

At the end of a string of hard days I was feeling particularly dumb. As in, 'pack your bags you're done', dumb. So, when I got home I immediately listed out the things that week I had done well, because Lord knows all the stuff I had done poorly needed some counter-action in my brain.

Sadly enough, I was not looking to prevent collapse of my patient under the weight of a disease process. It was not about saving a patient at all.
I was hoping to prevent my own collapse under the pile of fear, what-ifs, newbie nerves and lethal scenarios that I was conjuring in my head. I didn't want to be afraid of this new career I loved.

So, Nurse Awesome, there is just no way to talk about the first months of your nursing career without addressing the fears that are going to be running around in your head.

As non-glamorous as it is; fear is a big player as you move away from the protection of your professors and preceptors.

No matter what kind of hotshot you were in school.

Brace yourself; fear will dress itself in all kinds of fancy clothes. What it looks like does not matter. The result it produces is our only concern and the reason we are chatting about it straight away.

(Note to Self: Awesome nurses are not without fear; they simply do something proactive to deal with it. Just like we anticipate our patients' issues and do something about them up front. We are going to anticipate there will be fear and take great care of ourselves.)

Here's the bottom line, amazing face; fear makes you smaller than you are; it contracts you and that keeps you from sharing all of your best parts with the world.

Fear also keeps you from being the beneficial presence your patient needs you to be. It makes you hesitate beyond the healthy time it takes to run through a procedure in your head before you perform it. It paralyzes you and this makes for a sucky nurse. You do not have time for it.

Don't waste time hiding here; we all get scared from time-to-time. It is one of those elements of humanness that we cannot escape. Shit will hit the fan sometimes. Bad things will happen. Patients will die. You're gonna feel it. You don't have to let it paralyze you, though.
Being proactive and spending a bit of time examining what scares you can make an impact on just about everything.

- The outcome of your first year
- The way you craft your practice
- The way you view your role in the lives of your patients
- The way you move into the future once you find yourself standing on the other side of this first year

That is really just a short list of stuff that depends on you dealing with your fears sooner rather than later in this game.

I know that at least some part of you is scared pant less by the thought of working without the protection of nursing school, your professors, or the net labeled: I am just a 'student' nurse.

It is normal and it is not needed. Fear takes up space in both head + heart that could be filled with other things. You get to choose whether you keep it!

I was on the job a month, max, when I saw something I never expected. It showed how much power fear had to stop me. I was giving report to oncoming nurse when a bloody body ran smack into the glass door in front of me blocking entrance to the room.

Holy Shit! I was right in front of them, closest to helping. Although my mind said,' I need to do something now', my body did not move. No amount of NCLEXy-critical thinking scenario days in school prepared me for this scene. I slow-motioned it towards the door knowing I needed to take action but being paralyzed by fear instead.

There were many things in my head that needed doing now all of which were superseded by 'You are a new nurse you know nothing' screaming in my head! Fear caused me to shrink away from the experience and had stopped my brain at 'stop the bleeding'. The experienced nurses around me descended on this room like ants on an open candy bar.

Quickly, 3 of them pushed hard on the door wedging it enough for a super skinny gal to get in and hold pressure, check LOC and breathing status. Someone brought a backboard to get them off the ground, another threw towels on the puddle of blood, someone moved the bed closer to the patient, and another gal was checking the airway while still another hollered they were getting IV supplies since they had pulled out the central line. Still another person was on the phone with the ICU doctor and another was pulling medication they anticipated the doctor would order to sedate and intubate crazy blue and bleeding person. Even the rounding internal medicine doctor jumped in to help. Me? I just stood back and watched the gorgeous ballet of chaos the nurses around me danced.

I missed it because I was afraid. I missed it because I doubted my ability to be helpful as a new nurse.

Don't get me wrong, I learned a ton just from watching them work however; I also kicked myself in the ass fairly hard after the fact for not being in the middle of the action.

I let fear stop me. I let fear win.

I am going to make you this promise, amazing face.

I promise that the nurse you are today, as you emerge from school, looks nothing like the nurse you will be a year after you start your first nursing job. No duh, huh?

You didn't really need a book to tell you that, I know.

But in a way, you do need a book to tell you that because

school makes us into super-focused nursing machines that expect perfection in each step; a model which does not resemble real-life one single bit.

Only time helps you release the hesitation that you feel as a new nurse. If you look at your fears, acknowledge them and take a minute to reframe them you will move more quickly past the ones that halt you. You will begin to see the significance of your role and gain the confidence you see those experienced phenoms sporting all around you. Quickly.

That all sounds well and good, right? But Melissa, you ask, how EXACTLY are we gonna move from the place we are in now (afraid) to that place we want to be (unafraid)?

The exercises we chatted about in this chapter are a great start. Once you have those on lock we are going to use one of the cornerstones of our nursing practice and a few other simple bits to keep honing our craft.

Focus Point: Fear is hardly ever based on something in the present moment. We get afraid because of something that happened in the past (meaning it is over)or that might happen in the future (meaning it has not happened).

You can do nothing to change either of those things, you know? Deal with your fears as they come up and they will help you become a better nurse rather than cripple your patient care. You have a lot of information to assimilate in the months ahead as you start your first nursing job.

Action Step: Do not decide that you suck as a nurse based on the first few weeks of your real-world job. This stuff is tough. You are tougher.

Mantra Mojo: Put this on repeat in your head. Say it over and over until you feel strong. *I will not give my power to my fear.*

Come on Nurse Awesome, say it with me…

I will not give my power to my fear
I will not give my power to my fear
I will not give power to fear!

Dear Awesome New Nurse.

You look great in that new uniform. LOVE your new shoes, too!

You worked so hard in school to get to this place. It is a sweet spot you might not feel for a while so please stop and just absorb all that you have done in the last few years to get here.

Damn, you are awesome!

Love
Me

Shock + Awe

Your first patient experience with your new RN credential is going to put a huge smile on your face.

"Hi! My name is Melissa and I will be your nurse today..."

No lie, I rehearsed that line thousands of times during the years that finally produced those Registered Nurse credentials.

It was a powerful mantra. I believe words carry a great deal of power so I used these few, repeated often as part creative force, part affirmation and probably part mind-game in order to keep focus through all the late night study sessions, early morning clinical dates and assorted other redundant + ridiculous tasks that nursing school requires. It was especially useful when school felt more like a test of my ability to 'be flexible' than a place I was learning how to be a nurse.

Of course, along with the words came the myriad of daydreams about my first 'real job' nursing. I imagined myself a modern-day Florence Nightingale, able to fix broken bones +weary souls with ease while making a lasting impact on all my patients.

In my head I was the goddess of patient care.

You've no doubt had this day dream at least once. You know the one. Your hard-won pharmacology knowledge couples perfectly with your care planning prowess to kick some disease process ass, right?

In that space I know exactly what to say to patients to soothe their souls. Talking to doctors, pissed off patients, and angry families?

No sweat, because I am also a perfect therapeutic communicator. I could also insert a Foley Catheter, start difficult IV's and give medications no one could pronounce along with all the pertinent teaching without missing a step. I could dress a central line or drop an NG tube in minutes. I was organized, efficient and had perfect timing when it came to meeting the needs of both my patients and my peers.

You had at least one daydream where you were this superhero while you were in school, right?

While obviously daydreams, I told y'all I believe in the power of positive thought so while I was busting tail in school, I truly felt like the stuff going on in my head would easily reveal itself once I earned the title of Registered Nurse.

I had built up some serious nursing chops via countless hours in lab and had performed all those skills on real-live people. I had a high GPA + graduated with honors from a nationally recognized program. I naively believed the credentials to practice were the only missing piece.

I mean, come on, aside from school I have 'nursed' folks all my life and I suspect you have done the same. Actually passing my NCLEX meant that now I would get a paycheck for something I did naturally every day. Who wouldn't be excited about that, huh?

Sadly, positive thinking and all, the best part of my first week on the job was getting my name badge that said I was now officially an RN. I told everyone I met, 'Hey! I am an RN now!' I even wore my new name badge to the store. I was so happy + proud.

Other than that high point I spent a lot of time with my head cocked to one side like a curious dog, wondering what world I just stepped into, cause lord knows, it was not the one I spent 2 years prepping for in school.

I have 2 words for those first weeks in my new career:

Shock + Awe.

Come to find out, my understanding of what actually happens in a typical day of this noble calling was not much like the real deal. Even the time I spent in clinical did not prep me for what I experienced.

The workload placed on nurses, the knowledge you are expected to have from day one, the importance of the role, and the intensity of even the small actions barely scratched the surface of all I had in store for me or all I still had to learn despite all the school I had just completed.

I was in awe of how the seasoned vets maneuvered around all the hurdles placed in front of them and my God, were there ever a shit ton of hurdles.

The first few days I got to actually say "I am your nurse today" filled me with a panic that I cannot find words to describe.

No lie.

There was simply no way I could see myself ever being able to negotiate everything I saw the amazing nurses around me doing with ease.

I actually had a well-meaning soul tell me that I was only having an issue because I was working in an intensive care unit. My ego wanted to believe it.

Truth is that the first months of practice are hard regardless of the type of nursing you landed within.

It boils down to this; every single action you take matters. Every single can you take can harm or heal.

Even the actions you fail to take can harm or heal.

Every single time a human places their life in your hands it is powerful and potentially overwhelming.

Different areas of nursing will experience that differently, sure, however; every life matters.ICU, Medical, Oncology, Mother-Baby.

Dealing with life and death doesn't change as your area of practice changes. That is some heavy stuff, no?

I'd of never made it through nursing school if my daydreams had been rooted in even a tiny bit of reality or any one of the 50 million varieties of fear I was conjuring in my brain.

Thank goodness I didn't know any better in school.

There were some great days sprinkled among the ones that left me ragged. Smiley happy days were not the norm. Not that I allowed anyone to see that, of course. I kept my overwhelm strictly to myself.

Let me share what my first few weeks were like, okay?

Understand up front that I never once considered that I was leaving school 'unprepared' for the real world of nursing.

I loved the critical care world and still, at least 10 times a day; I felt I'd made a huge mistake leaving my corporate gig for this insanity. I reckoned I would either maim someone or create a sentinel event related to my inexperience.

It was a super-scary place to be in as a new nurse.

I was sitting in shift change around my 3rd week as an RN contemplating how to bridge the Grand Canyon sized gap when my inner awesome whispered to me: 'Look sweet pea;

32

there is nothing wrong with you. There is just a huge difference between the words qualified and prepared that you didn't factor in here.'

Thank GAWD it spoke up. I was bordering on breakdown.

It made sense.

The books I stayed buried in for two years + the shiny new license technically 'qualified me' but I was in no way 'prepared' for the decisions, juggling, and intensity of the real deal.

All the Code Blue lab days in the entire world did not make my adrenaline surge the way the real thing did.

My brain was on such overload that even something as simple as a different brand of normal saline shook me.

Look, I am not even joking.

I was so freaked out I would make a mistake that at the end of one particularly harsh day I looked at a bag of saline 10 times and actually asked my preceptor to confirm that 0.9% was the correct bag of normal saline for the order. Simply because the writing on the bag was blue rather than the black I was used to seeing.

Don't judge. I am aware that is pathetic.

I am sharing because you do not have to go to this place in your brain. You can reel-in a ton of freak out before it happens simply by knowing that at some point it will happen. I want you to dog-ear this page. If you get to that melt-down-holy-shit-i-suck-and-my-whole-life-is-over place come back and reread the long paragraph that follows:

Grab some popcorn while I layout the play-by-play in my *brain* those first weeks:

> What the heck is that disease, what is THAT test he ordered and why have I never heard of it? OMG, what the hell is a HELLP patient doing in ICU, I thought I would never have exposure to OB here. Odd, that symptom doesn't fit with that disease; I need to look that up. What does it mean again when there are tall peaked T waves? Is that my ventilator alarming? What buzzing alarm is that going off? Did I set the bed alarm? Was that a grimace I saw on their face, are they in pain or do they need more sedation? What is the difference anyway, pain med will sedate, right? Wait, BP is already in the tank if I give them morphine they will vasodilate and get an even lower pressure. Oh yea, maybe I can't do an accurate neuro check because of that so maybe they need less sedation? Which thing is most important here, I studied prioritization for heaven's sake! Where does this rank in Maslow's? Why didn't NCLEX test THIS SHIT? Why won't she stop pooping so much and why didn't school teach me how to keep it from running down the bed? What was the half-life of dilaudid again? Should I give this Valium so close to that dose of morphine, surely the doc wouldn't leave that as an option if it would harm my patient? Hydralazine or labetelol first for high BP? Is the Tylenol in Norco enough to decrease the fever of my patient or do I give a Tylenol suppository too? Will dilaudid and xanax and morphine suppress their respirations too much? Wait they are vented is that totally dumb to think that suppressing respirations is relevant? Holy cow, how am I supposed to be in 10 places at once? No human could ever do this long term. Why am I so

far behind? Why is the family asking these things, where is the doc? Where is that flow sheet at in the chart again? Oh Crap, I forgot to mark that chest tube drainage this hour, where did I write down that urine output number? How the heck do these restraints fit? I have to pee, I have not eaten, my feet hurt like king-hell, I need to chart, and it simply cannot be midnight already!

Pretty scary, huh?

You should have been in my head the first time a neurosurgeon asked me to assist him drill a burr-hole in someone's skull at the bedside and set-up the drain for it during my fourth shift ever as a nurse.

Yes, Nurse Awesome, you read this correctly. My fourth shift.

Ever. If I could insert ominous and terrifying music here I would…

It was wholly terrifying and not something we learned in school.
The truth of it was that all that school aside; I had no clue what my role in the big picture of the day was let alone for this specific procedure. My preceptor standing at the desk nodding her confidence in my ability to help was not helping me at ALL. Good thing the unit educator walked by the room and offered to gather supplies. Wouldn't you know, I forgot ~~many~~ most of the things the doctor needed for the procedure until I was gowned up and the whole scene was sterile, cause I am awesome that way!

I would've preferred to have been dropped at the bottom of the Grand Canyon on a July afternoon with no water and told to find my way up.

I was mentally, physically, and emotionally exhausted at the end of shift. All of them it seemed.

I don't mind telling you that I spent a little time being ticked off about it. Seriously, why had my instructors failed to teach me all this 'stuff'? I trusted them to prepare me **fully.**

I gave them my money and time and I worked my tail-end off with the promise that I would be ready to be a nurse. Dagnabit, it seems that somewhere sandwiched in all those damn therapeutic communication lectures or power points they didn't even test me on they would have mentioned at least *some* of this crap, right?

Their idea of teaching me organizational and critical thinking skills was not slightly applicable here. Good lord, what did I just spend all those hours learning anyway?

I felt like I was starting day one of school every single shift.

The only glimmer of hope those first weeks was when I recalled some fact about a disease process or medication that the super-nurses around me had long since filed under ' no longer needed' inside the computer-like nursing brain of theirs.

The first time I had to clean a patient you'd of thought the heavens had opened up and smiled on me, at least this was a task I was confident performing. Again, I am aware this is pathetic.

There are going to be stressors coming at you at a fast clip.

The speed at which I was being asked to make choices caused me to be a pretty hot-mess of insecurity which caused me to question everything I already knew about patient care, disease process and all other things nurse-ish.

One day, walking to my car post-shift I had this overwhelming thought, 'Damn, I suck at this; I am never going to be a nurse!'
Without my nursing buddy around for backup I sent out a plea to the heavens, 'For fuck's sake already, does every single day have to be so intense?!'

I instantly heard the same freaked out part of me laugh with a big fat, 'Yes, darlin, saving lives IS intense, these are NOT lab dummies. You ARE new to this craft so you WILL mess up.

What part of all THAT did you EXPECT would be easy?'

It was just the jolt of reality that I needed in that moment.

It took another 2 months of jolts plus quite a few internal bitch sessions before I fully realized that it was my own thoughts that were causing my biggest issues.

Say Whhhhhaaaaaatttt?

Yea, it was me. The expectations that I brought with me to the party did not match reality but overachiever that I am, I kept trying to make them match and when I failed in doing that I simply decided it was me that sucked; I didn't see any other possible explanation.

Enough about the suck y'all, let's talk about simple thought patterns you can change to remove the suck from this part of your life and your nursing practice.

1. I expected that I learned enough in school to know the ins and outs of the daily work of nurses to be able to slip right into the flow of the day and keep up with everything from day one. When I held this belief up to the light of day it showed itself as being totally unrealistic. Reframing was in order. I needed

to understand and accept that school was only the foundation for my practice. The beginning not the end, you know? I had been awesome at managing my time and workflow as a student however; there was much I still needed to learn about RN time management + work flow.

2. I was measuring my daily performance against that morphed up Florence Nightingale + experienced nurse vision from my daydreams. I thought I should be THAT kind of awesome already. I was expecting that I could jump right in and be as awesome as the incredible and experienced nurses on my unit. I surmised that having mastered care plans and clinical and having a high GPA and conquering NCLEX would translate to awesome nurse from day one. Wrong.

3. I thought asking for help or admitting I was overwhelmed was a sign of weakness.
I expected my peers to consider my asking for help as admission that I sucked. I could see my new peer group anticipating complicated connections between disease and symptom and what they needed to do about it then call the doc and suggest a course of action and I somehow thought that I should be able to do the same from the jump. Again, I was wrong.

4. I set a super-high bar from myself. Super-useful for school when everything you did was measured against a similar high bar, just not so useful in real-life. I needed to establish a new baseline. I needed to do that because this was not school. I needed to do this because I could not gain 20 years experience in 20 days. Without a new bat I was going to go crazy.

Get my drift, Nurse Awesome?

I was not an experienced student any longer.

I was a brand new nurse. The two are totally different things. There was no way that at this point in time I could be as good as the peers around me that made it look so darn easy.

The naked truth? It wasn't even easy for them. They have not cracked some magic code that unlocked amazing nursing superpowers. They have walked in your exact steps. They have already fumbled through learning time management and workflow. They have been hit in the head by enough curve balls that they look for them coming so they can duck. They have enough experience that they make plans based on the challenges that they can see are coming that you cannot.

Their superpowers have taken time to find.

That is all. You will get there, it just takes time.

Time is not something that an impatient new nurse has an excess of, right?

We want to be them now. We actually believe our patient population needs us to be them now. You know, with that whole life vs. death thing hanging over us it seems reasonable enough. Really they are just thoughts we need to adjust if we are to keep ourselves out of the land of suck.

So stop here for a minute. Have a stretch. Grab some tea. Let it sink in that the reasons for your shock are mostly in your control.

Take a minute to examine your own expectations for your transition to practice.

What kind of nurse do you expect you will be from day 1?

Are you being realistic or like me, are you expecting perfection from yourself from day one?

Here is how I broke down the points above in a way that was 100 times more useful than my original thoughts.

1. Instead of just beating myself up for my inability to be in 'the flow' of my new role I became a student of the great nurses around me. I observed everything these brilliant people were doing for their patients and I copied it as consistently as I could manage. I had to let go of some of my student habits that were not serving me and incorporate some new ones however; that was easy enough. Now, you do the same. Observe what you see around you and take notes on the actions and words of the nurses on your unit that exhibit the skills you admire. Whether that is actually patient care of something as simple as they way they organize their room. Once you get your head firmly wrapped around the thought that experienced student nurse and experienced nurse are different things you will be able to cut yourself some slack and get on with more positive things.

2. Let's be real, most of us learned in school to be horribly harsh on ourselves when it comes to anything related to our nursing practice. School builds this into us on purpose-cause life vs. death, you know? Keep in mind that there is a whole new skill set to learn here, Nurse Awesome. For example, starting an IV on someone in school lab is a simple task. Add to that the patient who is terrified of pain jerking his arm back every time you approach his skin, this adds a level of difficulty you can't get until you get to the

real-world. So this is another one of those areas that you get through quickly if you observe the nurses around you that you admire.

3. Allow yourself to ask for help, please. It really is okay. I know, I know. It goes against the dog-eat-dog world of school that says you'd better know everything + you better be perfect at it. This world is vastly different than school in many ways and this is one of them. It is okay to say, 'I need help, I really don't understand or I really feel overwhelmed or whatever.' Sadly, most of us leave school with this bogus belief that we will be killed or fired or shamed if we admit there is something we don't know. I swear though, it is just the opposite. The other people on your floor know that you are new and that you will need help. Give yourself permission to be supported instead of always having to appear strong and together. Ask before you take action if at all possible. Wait until you mess up is not always the best course of action. Trust me here; they already know you need help so just get it when you need it. This was a particularly hard area for me to master. Asking for help felt to me like advertisement of ignorance. That was my ego and a lot of old stories in my head talking. By the way, hyperventilation at the nurses' station does not actually qualify as asking for help, speak up!

4. Enough with the perfection thing. It is not an attractive quality in a nurse. The full court press for perfection was not healthy for me at all. It will not be healthy for you. Expecting yourself to be as efficient and effective as the experienced nurses around you...well, it will make you nuts. Knowing you will mess up yet feeling like you cannot ever mess up will fill you with anxiety. Just don't go here. I walked into many shifts the first month feeling horrible about myself before I even started. I know you are thinking that you would never expect yourself to be perfect. It

41

seems like a dumb thing, doesn't it? When you start dreading going into your shift regroup and come back to this place. You probably don't want to go into work for some reason that touches on how imperfect you feel. Allow yourself to be imperfect.

Plenty of things will give you stress right now so, steer clear of the self-imposed variety. These are all things you can control.

Isn't that excellent news?

When our internal quest for awesomeness couples up with our unrealistic beliefs there is not any way we can succeed. They set us up to fail.

Realize this and you will be able to recognize this mind-gamey crap as it is happening from your first day in the real-world rather than 6 months into your practice as you sob on the way home from work every day feeling like the biggest loser-nurse in the history of ever.

I promise that you are not even close to that being that nurse. Project neither doom and gloom nor perfection into your brand new nursing practice.

View this time as a transition. Allow yourself the time to put one toe at a time in the information flood rather than throwing yourself in and being drowned by it.

How are you supposed to do that, you ask? Well it is simple, it is just not easy given the preconceived notions we carry around.

In a nutshell you just set your intention to do it, then go and do it!

This will make it easier- Start your day with this simple intention. Call it a focus point or a magic spell. I don't care.

Let it serve as a reminder. Let it be the pair of floaties saving you from drowning in fear. Even if you think it sounds like the cheesiest thing ever (many of the left-brained people reading this will think that exact thing).

Do it anyway. Write it down and put it in your pocket then read it before each shift, during shift and after shift. Really.

On this day in each moment...
>I will show myself the same compassion I show to my patients.
>I will act with integrity + passion; always
>I will accept that I am not ever going to be perfect.
>I will mess up + that is okay; I am here to learn.
>I will feel overwhelmed + that will get better in time.
>I will use each event in my day to consciously craft my practice.

Trust me. Even if you think I am off my rocker. Say it for 30 days, every day without fail. It will help you to anchor realistic expectations. It will set intention for each day and it will help you remember that you are *new* nurse, not a PERFECT nurse.

There will be days that no matter what action you take you still feel less than warm + fuzzy about your ability, your job, your choice to a nurse in the first place. Pay attention to how you are feeling. When you recognize some suck(aka fear) coming on do something different to correct and release the feeling.

I use mantras like the one above a lot to course correct myself. I don't much care if my co-workers think I am insane when they hear me whispering to myself. They work for me.

I consider them little petitions to the Universe for help as well as reminders to myself of how I want to feel or what I want to experience in my life. I use them in my nursing to keep from feeling overwhelmed and to refocus once I get overwhelmed. They help me stay grounded in the things that matter to me.

I typically start my shift with the above mentioned focus point and then, as I get out of my car and start to head in the building I recite some version of this little mantra.

I am an amazing and capable RN. I know my hands are guided to take the best action for each patient and I am a force for good to all I encounter.

It changes depending on how I feel and I say it to myself at least 20 times a day. When I first started it was more like 50 because I felt overwhelmed a lot! Plus, when I first started I felt like asking to be led to take the best action for each patient was the perfect prayer. It relieved a ton of stress for me. Try mine and see what you think or make up a version all your own. In some way, remind yourself that you are not alone, that you have some control in the seemingly craziness of new nurse land and that you want to focus on the positive of your day.

For reasons unknown to me, these simple adjustments were like magic. Realigning my expectations of my ability as a new nurse and actually asking for help when I needed it; brilliant! Setting a bar I could actually reach on the daily, setting the intention that I was going to have a good shift and then using my simple mantra in order to help me course correct. Exactly the kind of empowering that I needed.

I am not kidding. Once my perspective shifted + I gave myself a break from the 'perfection expectation' I spent a lot less time feeling like a failure.

So, Nurse Awesome, are there things you need to adjust?

Are you expecting that you will be perfecto as you make the transition from student to nurse? How can you allow yourself to be supported while maintaining the confidence level needed to provide awesome patient care?

If you can let go of the need for perfection in just one area, what area would pick?

The voice in your head that says you are supposed to know it all is an asshole. You will see huge change in your transition to practice once you can tell it to shut the hell up.

The people that hired you know you are new and that your awesomeness is a work in progress and this is really exactly the place to be.

Once I was able to show my lack of confidence and ask for help it was easier to start measuring my performance against my own performance instead of the wonderkins around me. What a relief to not have to be perfect all the time.

Another funny thing happened, too. When I showed vulnerability they did too. Some of them told me they admired my encyclopedia-like knowledge of all things anatomy or that they wished they could do things like me. Total shocker.

It was good to know that even experienced nurses are sometimes scared shitless in the middle of a code. It was a relief to know that few of those nurses I admired had ever assisted a neurosurgeon drill burr holes at bedside so they would have also been unsure, like me. What??? I never considered that any of them would be unsure of anything at this point in their careers.

There is such depth to your new nursing gig that you cannot

learn everything in school. There is just no way on earth that school can expose us to all of it.

Remember, school is just the foundation, right?

That means start...you learn as long as you are a nurse.

Remember, this is a nursing *practice*, not a nursing *perfect*.

Experience helps to minimize your missteps however as long as you are human you will be prone to messing up sometimes.

You cannot get completely free from fear + stress during the first months. You worked your buns off to get here. You endured many a long night and many a crazy NCLEX question to earn that license. Being attached to having a good outcome is natural. Wanting to do an excellent job is natural. Setting a high bar is all good...you can do all that and not kill yourself in the process.

Focus Point: Examining the expectations you hold for yourself as you transition into like as an RN and adjusting your expectations and setting reasonable goals will give a much different results than demanding perfection will. Once I got this piece straight I was able to get in a better head space quickly. I was able to sleep and feel like I was a contributing member of the team, despite my lack of 'worldly-nursing-knowledge.'

Action Step: Develop a ritual to let go of your mistakes. Get in the habit of releasing stress through physical activity. Forgive yourself for imperfection. Allow yourself to be human.

Mantra Mojo: The time I took to set my intention for the day and work out my own personal helpful mantra helped to create a positive space which has only fed more positive.

Start with this and add words that make you feel confident and strong.

I am an amazing and capable RN:

It took me a minute to get past the hokieness here. Once I actually used some mantras in my nursing practice to help me focus and remember who I am under all that shock and awe of the first few weeks I discovered they really do were worth the time investment. They have been a win-win...for me, my peers and my patients
.

Feeling a little more empowered, Nurse Awesome?

Good!

Now, there is another tool that we can use that will empower you in these first months of practice even further.

You don't really even have to learn something new. You have been doing this throughout school. Let's explore...

Dear Buttercup~

Just wanted to remind you that fear is a liar +
you can choose to believe it or not, ya know?

It would be especially wise not to change
everything in your life and give up on a
lifetime dream when you are exhausted and
hungry and your feet are killing you. Rest
first, please.

Take a minute and regroup yourself. Don't worry
about all the potentially insane and crazy
situations the day might bring. Your incredible
peer group has your back; I promise they will not
let you kill anyone.

Take a breath…now isn't that better.

You have everything you need to succeed
already inside you, of course you know that
already!!!

Love Beyond the Moon~

Me

HONEST SELF ASSESSMENT

Yep, as simple as it sounds, it is the ticket outta fear-town for new nurses! Good thing it is also a skill we've spent years in school perfecting, huh?

Assessment is the cornerstone of everything for nurses.

A great assessment can mean the difference between life + death for your patient. It can mean the same for your career; thorough self-assessment creates a solid foundation on which to build the rest of your practice.

By using your mad assessment skills, the first months of your new job can move from something you fear to something that kicks 1000 kinds of ass.

Our first activity each shift revolves around assessing our patient.

It is first because it is important! We need to get the skinny on those things that need the focus of our care, what we should do first and what can wait until later in the shift.

While we take report from another nurse and get the down-low on what has been going on for that patient throughout *their* shift remember that this information is given to you through someone else's nursing brain filter; not your own.

While important, it is information that lives in the past.

It's '**what-was,** not **what-is'** going on with your patient. It is someone else's analysis of what the patient needs. While the best nurses listen to + collaborate with other nurses they also always trust what they see, hear, and feel for themselves above another's interpretation of a patient condition.

Awesome nurses take action on intel that they
gathered, not based on data someone else collected.

Same is true for your nursing practice. It is good to listen
to the guidance of the people that came before you
however; f you approach your first year of nursing based
on your personal inadequacies as seen through the eyes
of someone else you will still feel lost a year in. If you
passively accept a 'plan of attack' that someone else
created for you without your own insight into what you
need then it will give you a ton of grief and cause you to
work harder than you have to in order to get your
bearings.

Follow me here. How can someone else be in your mind and
know what is making you afraid, paralyzed, sleepless,
confused, cranky + closed up?

Well, they can't really now can they, right?

Nope they cannot. So, don't spend your time being afraid of
a skill or patient situation because someone _else_ thinks you
should be afraid.

Don't try to fit your practice into a box that someone else
says is a 'good practice'. Don't hold yourself up next to
someone with 20 years experience and judge your progress
on it. If you compare yourself or your own nursing practice
to others, then you will be disappointed + frustrated a lot.

This will not feel awesome.

You have to take some time and look at what is or is not
happening for you. Just you.

That's why this book is not a step-by-step, 'must-do'
workbook. There are no 'musts, there is only what works for
you.

It's why I will ask you to check in with your own wisdom rather than relying solely on my version of what is best for you.

Check this out, Nurse Awesome.

Without doing it intentionally, school sets us up for trouble here. It dumps us in a group and then compares us to one another in many of the tasks we are given. It homogenizes us because that is how it can most easily measure performance of a mass of people. It compares us to standards because we need to be safe in our practice and must be able to meet the criteria the governing agencies set not because that is how we should continue measuring ourselves once we get out into the real-world.

It's the path of least resistance after so much school comparison for you to immediately compare yourself to the other nurses on your floor.

Naturally, after being in an environment that compared you as the norm, you are going to compare yourself. When you do that and you see that you are nowhere near 'the same' as those other nurses you will start to freak out a bit. Never mind that your measuring yourself next to someone that has 10 more years in the field than you, you will think that your performance is horrible next to your experienced peers.

Listen up. Dump the comparisons. You're out of school now and you have a chance to create a practice that focuses on your unique talents and strengths.

Hoorah!

You will adhere to a set of standards of course and provide evidence-based care. It is just that you get to express yourself between those lines once you establish some basics of care.

You get to decide what type of nurse you want to be, you get to decide which of your best parts you want to focus on in the care you provide. Kindness is important to me so in the middle of all that evidence-based care I choose to find ways to express it in all areas of my shift. Integrity or procedural knowledge might be 'your' focus point so you might find ways to focus on that rather than kindness. You see, it is up to you what type of nurse to be, isn't that amazing after being 'told' how you have to be for all that time in school? Man, it was for me!

Here's the rub, though. Without some self-assessment the things you believe to be the most beneficial about your presence will not come from you at all; they will come from instructors, friends, other nurses who know nothing about you.

It will feel a little like trying to squeeze into someone else's jeans. The fit is just not right and while you may be able to do it short term you cannot sustain it long-term. You can't be the nurse someone else believes you are over the course of an entire career.

Plus, you will not be able to look back a year from now and see how far you came because you started with someone else's baseline assessment of where you were at in the first place.

Self-assessment is really about finding the place that stops your flow of inner awesome. When that stops you cannot sustain a feeling of commitment and joy around your new profession. In doing this we are going to be working with the tasks that give you jitters so you can gain confidence plus defining the things you already rock at doing so that you can do those things more often; further building your confidence, phenom.

For me it was about finding the place that was open and confident rather than closed and afraid. Taking the time to do this kinda helped me lean into that space on a deeper level, which helped me to start to really love what I do each day; even on those days when there is little on the surface to love. Even more, for me, it was about finding the intersect between smart and big-hearted. Things I consider my best parts.

What do you consider your best parts, Nurse Awesome?

It takes a little work to do a good self-assessment. You have to look at yourself over a period of days or weeks to create a great plan of care that supports your awesomeness however; it is amazing how much this simple thing will empower you.

If you take the time to do this I swear to you that your feelings about your transition to practice will change.

Open and 'in the flow' feels so much better than 'closed and out of the flow.' As we move forward into this place keep these things in mind, okay?:

Your patient is dynamic; the issues + needs change throughout the day so they deserve individual attention not a cookie-cutter approach AND you and your nursing career are no different; dynamic + deserving of individual attention.

Let's look at ourselves with a critical eye, so we can diagnose the things that may give us grief and make a plan to change them, to circumvent them and to prevent them. This does not have to be hard or time consuming.

Start simple. Take a minute at the end of each shift and ask yourself these simple questions.

What skills or situations did I feel super-comfortable performing? Write that down (**Note to self**: no, you will not remember it so write it down!)

What skills or situations made me feel not so great? Write these down, too. What skills did I have no idea how to perform?

Write them down. What equipment was I unfamiliar with on my floor? Write, write, write...

Don't leave out the psychosocial situations, skills, basic theory stuff, pharmacology; all of it. (**Note to Self**: Psych stuff is important!)

Was I comfortable talking with patients about end-of-life issues?

Did I hit the vein quickly or fumble with the IV start kit still?

Did I know the disease process my patient was fighting and what sort of care I should be providing them based on that disease? You get the drift here I am sure.

I kept a blank index card in my pocket to scribble on as each shift went along; in fact, I still do it two years later. *(Note to Self:* Ongoing self-assessment is a habit of awesome nurses).

Here is my verbatim list from the index cards I carried my first week (seriously):

Melissa's Tools for Becoming Nurse Awesome

> <u>I rock at</u>: head-to-toe assessments, pharmacology, talking about hard shit, like dying and making pathophysiology simple for total strangers, calming

down demented people, redirecting negative chat, helping people see the good side in something that appears to only be bad.

I suck at : NG tube insertion on demented people, starting IV's on dehydrated people, the etiology + treatment of septic shock, getting meds from the Pyxis, making sure I know where the crash cart is at so I can help my patient quickly, telling the difference between v-tach and interference from movement.

Based on this list can imagine what that week was like?

The next week's list was different. I learned some new drugs that week, added rectal tubes on combative patients to the 'I suck at list' and corrected my lack of knowledge of equipment storage.

So, remember that comparison thing I told you not too long ago was bad for you? I did this with gusto when I finally got my own license.

Of course, I work with some incredible nurses so that left me with a heavy 'I will never be good enough' complex by week twos end.

I spent a couple of hard nights beating myself up over that "I suck at" list until one day, mid-shift, I brought my preceptor a drug that was scheduled to be given but that I felt should be held. I wanted to talk to Doctor Awesome before giving it because I thought the current lab values of the patient, the age/co-morbidities of the patient and the metabolism/excretion of the drug were gonna be a bad combination. She did not see the same issue as I did but allowed me to ask the doctor about it anyway. I explained my rationale and guess what; I was right, he corrected the MAR and thanked me for my diligence.

Say whhhaaattt? I could hardly believe it and neither could my preceptor. She encouraged me to 'enjoy my fresh from school brain' while it lasted. <insert huge smile here>

All I could focus on was that I actually knew something. I knew one small thing, in a sea of a bazillion things I had no clue about; my action was beneficial.

This meant so much to me. I needed that boost of confidence in my own brain. It showed me how important it was to trust my gut instinct and most important it showed me that I did not actually suck at everything nursing. Huge because at that point I felt I did.

So onward now.

It makes sense that after you have done some self-assessment and found some things you could improve on that you would want to feed yourself a few tidbits of awesome, right?
Yep! That would be the next things to do here...

Find the thing you are good at then do that thing' a lot, right?

Based on my week 1 self assessment, I volunteered to take dying patients, demented patients; I ran all the pharm through my head for compatibility and actually taught the patients that were awake about what I was giving them.

Since practice makes you better all-around....

Find the thing you are not so good at and do it more.

Based on my week 1 self assessment I told everyone at report that I would insert all NG tubes and start any IV they would let me start. I printed out the rhythm strip each time the monitor alarmed with V-tach and examined it. I asked other nurses for their perspective. I learned the difference between equipment and patient failure quickly this way.

Yes, asking to do more of the stuff I sucked really did suck however; by the end of that first week I was feeling much more confident at all those things. I sucked a little less at them; even with a long way to go before I was a pro.

Confidence=open + happy nurse, right?

Lesson learned after that first week for me.

> *Do the things that you feel good and confident doing A LOT. Do the things you suck at even more.*

Make a list like this your first months and see what it tells you about your own skills? Make some plans to practice the things you are not so hot with a little more each week. Tell other nurses you feel you suck at these tasks and ask for help. Don't procrastinate + don't be afraid to look dumb to your peer group. They were all new nurses once and most of them will be happy to share their knowledge with you.

Fear, in a lot of cases as a new nurse, is just really a lack confidence, right?

Confidence comes with repetition so put yourself into situations intentionally which will in turn help decrease your fear, right?

It might suck but you build trust in your ability to survive and thrive in those situations by being in them not by shying away.

I STILL use this to strengthen my practice.

You should have seen the look on my co-workers face when I asked to be allowed to insert the rectal tube that was ordered and draw labs on their patient in a Rotoprone bed.

Hey, don't judge, some things you cannot learn until you get to do them and I had never inserted a rectal tube before nor worked on someone in a crazy bed like that one! I truly needed the practice!

No matter how long you nurse, practice is the only way to gain confidence, right?

This first year will be as unique as you.

It will not look the same as anyone else.

It is not supposed to, remember? We no longer want to homogenize ourselves or be exactly like anyone but us! Don't compare yourself with your school buddies.

Enough talk, let's figure out what you are good at right now by assessing the skills you bring to this table.

(Note to Self: don't freak out, there are tons of skills you didn't learn in school)

Let's peek at your hard skills

How confident are you that you could do these without 30 minutes to complete the task? Rate yourself on a scale of 1-10

IV starts _____
Getting a patient to the potty _____
Attaching 12 lead EKG lines _____
Setting up O2 for your pt _____

Assessing for skin issues _____
Blood Draws _____
Foley catheter insertion _____
NG Tube Insertion _____
Rectal Tube Insertion _____
CVP/Art Line Monitor Setup _____
Sterile dressing change _____

Are there some hard skills you'd rather not have to do at all?
Tell it here:

- _____
- _____
- _____
- _____
- _____
- _____
- _____

Are there some soft skills that you know you need to bone-up
on prior to your entry into Smiley General? Tell it here:

- _____
- _____
- _____
- _____
- _____

What scares the bajeezus outta you?

- _____
- _____
- _____
- _____
- _____
- _____

Now let's peak at those soft skills: What patient situations that are not <u>hard</u> skill related make you afraid/nervous? This is the time to let your fear run wild...

Rate yourself on a scale of 1-10 in these specific areas

Dying patients _____
Angry patients _____
Angry families _____
Demented patients _____
Needy patients _____
Drug seekers _____
Suicidal Patients _____
Newly diagnosed patients _____
Obese patients _____

What patient situations do you <u>know</u> you can handle without assistance? Come on, I know you have some, Nurse Awesome!

- _____
- _____
- _____
- _____
- _____
- _____
- _____

What do you expect this year to be like? Talk me through your expectations of a typical day in your job.

_____
_____
_____
_____

How do you expect to feel at the end of the day??

_____
_____
_____
_____

Remember a situation(s) in your nursing school that left you feeling awesome?

_____
_____
_____
_____

What specifically made you feel awesome about that situation?

_____
_____
_____
_____

What kinds of patient situations made you feel not so hot?

_____
_____
_____
_____

What was it about that situation that hurt you?

_____

_____

_____

_____

Was there a particular patient situation that touched you?

_____

_____

_____

_____

Tell me about that moment when you KNEW, 'Yep, I picked the right career!'

_____

_____

_____

_____

What things are most important to you that you include in your practice these first few months?

_____

_____

_____

_____

What fears or obstacles do you feel stand in your way of including them?

_____

_____

_____

_____

Now, use the tool on the next page for 3 shifts to record highs + lows and help you further assess yourself objectively.

For ease and accuracy of data capture write the columns on a note card, carry it in your pocket.

These points of focus will show you where you need work and more importantly they will show you were you are feeling confidence in your new role.

I'll ask again for you to complete this task even if you cannot see the value upfront.

This is the most important part of the assessment because it helps you build a realistic plan of attack that is as unique as you are.

You will be able to adjust that plan as you move through the first weeks of your job so don't waste tons of time trying to be prefect about this whole exercise. This is not school.

Try it...

I want you to keep some form of the chart that follows with you and tally it every single day. It helps to see both accomplishments and area to improve on in writing when your brain is frazzled. And it will be..

Today I Rocked At:	Today I Sucked At:

You have everything in you that you need to succeed in your new career.

You passed the NCLEX and you know how to find any info you may lack.
If you decide not to work through any of the other questions in this chapter please, use the Awesomeness Assessment above each day for 2 months .Practice what you need to practice and adjust your list accordingly. It will help you gain confidence and gain it quick..

More importantly though, the time you take to assess yourself will shine light on things you already kick-ass doing, so you can do more of those things.

If there is a magic wand that transforms your first year as a nurse into something that resembles what you have imagined it to be all those years in school, I believe that self-assessment is that magic wand.

It puts the power back in your hands by giving you direct access to your own skills and your own needs. It points to individual points of fear directly so you can address and correct them directly.

It does not rely on someone else's assessment of your nursing skills nor exaggerate your current knowledge base in any way.

Fear will not help you move forward because it closes you up. It places a box around your practice. It keeps you from exploring all the options + alternatives. It tells you big-fat-hairy-lies that keep you from growth. You don't need those limitations, magic face.

Keep your mind focused on doing things that open you up. I want you to spend this first year doing something beyond worrying about messing up the small stuff. Odds are, at some point you will, so just accept it and move on.

Don't wait on it; don't beat yourself up over it when it happens.

If you can get good + honest with yourself here and work through this self assessment you will see that what you are really doing is creating a rock solid foundation for your future.
You have to climb this 'first year' mountain anyway, you may as well empower yourself to show up in all your awesomeness instead of letting fear run the show, right?
Let's start thinking about making that transition to your first nursing job.

- What do you imagine the first few months in practice will be like for you? Spend some time in your head and create the day. Can you see the potholes in the daydream version of those first months?
- Do you know the difference between the skills you can + cannot do well? Do you know where you need help?
- Have you set a bar you can reach or do you expect yourself to be perfect? (**Note to self:** perfection is impossible)
- Do you have a realistic baseline for yourself? What are you most afraid of having happen?

The best way to step into your new career is to keep the excitement of being a nurse alive. What are you excited about going into this first job? Do you have an ego that is screaming at you that might keep you from asking for help? What can you do to quiet that ego?

A beginner's mind is not always a bad thing. Start to think about it as an asset rather than a liability.

A fresh, new mind is a gorgeous and powerful.

There is something you can do to resolve just about every situation that occurs no matter how new you may be to nursing. Just do not give up !

This fact alone can anchor you a bit and keep you from spinning into crazy town inside your head during these first few months of practice.

Let each day unfold without deciding up front what it will bring you. Just because yesterday sucked does not mean today will suck, too.

(Note to Self: Balance reality with enthusiasm,mmmk?) Enough with the self assessment.

Bottom line is that this first year is all about crafting your practice.

It is about building confidence + taking an active role in your own career. With the right tools on your superhero utility belt, well, it will be a hugely empowering year.

Doing an honest self-assessment and creating a plan to strengthen yourself where needed is not only empowering it is an incredibly easy way to build the confidence you need to show your inner-awesome

Focus Point: The points of tension for you on your first day will be things you laugh at a month into the journey. Your fears and confidences will change as you grow throughout your career. The things you love and hate will change. You will change.

Action Step: Go back and actually do the assessment.

Mantra Mojo*: I am an amazing person and I choose to*

consciously create my experience as I begin my nursing practice.

Put this mantra on repeat in your brain as you drive into work.

Now let's explore some other helpful bits for this first month of practice, Nurse Awesome.

ESSENTIAL ELEMENTS

A thorough self-assessment is the first part of the equation of awesome. There are a few other things you need to get in the habit of doing from day one of your nursing career. Without these bits of gold the earth will not stop spinning of course, BUT...in their absence you will spend more time with that something 'just doesn't feel right' space than is any fun and you don't need that feeling.

I was a good student + believed I would be a great nurse. Still, I felt totally unprepared nearly every day for my first month on the job. Trying to instill a sense of calm and confidence in your patient is hard when you are scatter-brained + scared.

That is what these essential elements help with; getting rid of the scatter-brained space. This is not a space you nurse well from, so spend some time with the focus points that are listed in the next 2 chapters to shorten your relationship with the yuck.

Oddly enough, none of the stuff in these chapters was taught directly in any of my school lecture hours or clinical times. I guess it was an assumed we would learn these things while on the floor during class.

These items are essential for your mental health as well as for your patients' physical health.

I am not trying to get all drama-queenish on you; I have just felt the difference they make so I want to inform you of the potential pothole. It is your choice to pay them any mind and use them or not.

They act as the foundation of your practice. They keep your patients safe and can accelerate your arrival to the comfy-spot in the new job space.

They will lay neatly right on top of that foundation you built through self-assessment and add to your sense of confidence.

With no further delay, the essential items I wish someone had chatted in depth with me about before I started working as a nurse are:

- Carrying the correct tools
- Setting up your room
- Getting to know your floor layout

Sounds simple enough? Powerful things usually are simple.

Note: Some of the information provided here will be specific to the patient and their disease. Some of it will be global; meaning it applies to each and every patient. Some specific to an ICU floor because that is where I trained. Please note this information is by no means all-inclusive. It is only a starting point. I will be the first to encourage you to find your own 'essentials' as you grow into your role through the first few months on shift.

Carrying the correct tools

This is an area that will probably change many times in your first few months. I lost a lot of pens in school so I was one of those freaks that started my first shift with 5 ink pens, a red pen and a pencil in my scrub pocket. I learned quickly that I needed that room for other things and I could stash extra pens in my bag or in the desk drawer if needed so I changed to a single multi-colored bic and a sharpie marker instead. The sharpie quickly moved from my pocket to behind my badge because I hated the thought of reaching into my pocket over + over with all those nasty cooties on my hands.

I also stuffed my pockets full of alcohol wipes in school. I started that way on my floor but quickly evolved into just a few of them with my 'stack' being in the room I was working in; and even then my stash was not big. We have carts outside each patient room were these are kept, again, saving room for more important stuff.

Spend some time the first few weeks and pay attention to what it is you need. Are you constantly fumbling with tight connections like me? You might need some hemostats. I never leave home without them now and they make my life so much easier.

Do you deal with a lot of orthopedic patients that have dressings you change? You may need some bandage scissors. If you are a neuro or an ICU nurse you will need a good penlight on the ready at all times. I started with one of these but quickly noticed that all the rooms on our floor keep a flashlight in them so that was one less thing attached to me.

If you are a cardiac nurse you cannot own enough hemostats in all sizes, I still have no idea what they are all for, I just know that all the CABG nurses on my floor plop a big wad of them down on the desk every shift.

I used to look like a hobo when I started my shift. Seriously, I had so much stuff 'stuffed' in my pockets I could barely sit down. Spending gobs of time rummaging through my pockets to find what I needed got old, fast.

Now I carry hemostats clipped to my scrub top by my pocket, trauma shears in my pants pocket along with a couple of flushes, a single ink pen in my scrub top pocket with a few alcohol wipes, a baby tin of breath mints, and my patient info sheet. My badge holds two colors of sharpie for marking IV bags and dressings, my keys to the med fridge and the PCA pump. It works well for me to keep my scrub top pockets as empty as possible for meds and the like so I only wear pants with pockets on the legs.

I know this sounds too simple but isn't it usually those simple items that make or break us? Spend a bit of time here once you've been on the floor a couple of weeks~

- What things are you always fumbling to find?
- What are you using most?
- What do you carry that you never use?

Change up what you carry and where you carry it on your person until it flows. You know you found the sweet spot when you find yourself not even thinking about where to grab it. Once you find that sweet spot then duplicate it over and over again. Habits are mind-savers in nursing. There is something to be said for always knowing where things are at when you need them.

Getting to know your floor layout

Seems like a no-brainer, huh? The first month you are on your floor, in your hospital orientation + preceptor time there will be a ton of information flying at you. The sheer amount of data you are expected to take in and then assimilate into working knowledge can paralyze you. There is no controlling the flood of info that is going to come at you so just take a breath and use your mad prioritization skills to figure out what you better know now and what you can spend some time remembering later.

(Note to Self: most of the stuff you don't need will be written down for you in a nice pretty orientation-type handout. The stuff you need flies out your preceptor's mouth at 100 mph.)

Getting to know the layout of your unit and your floor protocol for working a code should take priority over how to file your PTO requests or what fridge to use for your lunch. That is all I am saying.

I told you that I spent the first month with the yuck, right? A big part of my anxiety as a newbie came from a very generalized + unprepared feeling. I had it all the time and it took me a month to put my finger on it. I mean, I knew the hospitals mission statement to providing awesome patient care but I did not know where to access the tools that would help me keep those patients alive while demonstrating the behaviors management championed.

I walked into the shift each day feeling lost and like I had just stepped onto a foreign planet; totally alien.

I didn't know anyone, I didn't know where anything was located; I was constantly on the search for what I needed. I didn't understand the customs of the unit; I didn't know the language well. I had not yet learned the technical name for the billiontyleven gauze sizes or dressing types. It took me a minute to replace the word thingamajig with the medically correct name for tools I used, and it took even longer to learn Dr. Awesome's medication preference for central line insertions. The reason for their preferences, etomidate for intubations as opposed to versed and fentanyl for example, took me even longer to grasp.

I didn't know all the items needed in a procedure or what my role in that procedure was, so, I was constantly feeling like I was performing tasks in the dark, totally out of control.

Having just emerged from the world of school where organization is the key to survival it was no wonder I was stressed by all the not knowing and disorganization in my mind. I mean, the whole of it left me feeling a hair away from killing someone as a result.

Can you imagine how much stress that puts you under, seriously?

As a new nurse you pretty much live in flight or fight mode every shift for the first half a year so adding the stress of having to track something down in a true emergency was too much to handle.

I knew there were tons of people around me that I could ask for help but even that left me feeling like a newbie and amped my adrenaline to an unacceptable level, you know? Just don't do this to yourself, make it your goal in month one to learn where stuff is at on your floor.

It is not rocket science but no one on your floor is going to lead you by the hand to make sure you know. They may point it out to you on the grand tour of the place but knowing it is up to you.

(Note to Self: crash carts + artificial airway carts are tres importante so find them pronto.)

Where exactly is the code cart kept? Where is the emergency airway cart kept? Where is the code button on the wall? What is the procedure on your unit for calling a full code? How do you call for a rapid response team to come help you with a crashing patient? Who can you expect to come and help you? What is your role in all of it?

Learn this quick and know it cold. You will not have time or brain capacity to hunt and/or figure this out when your patient is coding.

PS..this is important info for every nurse, regardless of the floor.

Every single day for the first week, make it part of your daily chore to identify what room the crash cart is located next to on your unit. Look at it from the room you are in, plot how you will get it if you need it fast. Really, hunting sucks in a code, it is important to know even if your patient is on the more stable side of stable.
Go look at the plug situation on the back of the defib unit. Are pads kept attached to the defibrillation and heart monitor unit? If not, how will you get them fast?

If you have never seen inside this crash cart ask for a schematic or a lesson on the locale of things inside the cart from the person that restocks it. Make your way to the cart after it has been used and snoop a bit. Meds are usually on the top shelf but not always. Meds in a crash cart are packaged differently than from the Pyxis. No time to draw from a vial. You need to know how to dispense these meds and school may or may not have taught you.
Every single day of week two go to the supply Pyxis and determine the location of supplies you will use frequently or emergently.

True and miserably embarrassing story, my first week in ICU I was asked to get a Subdural Evacuating Port Kit and a Ventriculostomy Drain Setup by a neurosurgeon that just strolled in the room and decided we were going to do the procedure at bedside; right now. I had no clue where to find that stuff. Lucky for me when I entered the supply room one of those rock star nurses I worked with pointed them out of me, even luckier that the nurse educator was there to assist with what I forgot. Thank God for that, and thank God I knew it was out of my scope of practice to give an antibiotic thru the port....

I had a hard time shaking the feeling of 'you idiot' off me

when I left that day. It really brought into focus for me how lost I was over some simple things and how that all the hospital orientation had done nada to really prepare me to act quickly on my unit, you know? I was not on the quick path to being the ass-kicking nurse I envisioned.

So, I could have spent a lot of time beating myself up for the 'not-knowing' or chastising my unit peeps for having a crappy orientation.

Neither of those things would have addressed my issue though and it would have just left other people feeling bad and me sounding like a crazy gal, right?

Lucky for me, learning where stuff was at and what it was 'technically called' was a relatively easy area to gain some mastery over quickly. So I took personal responsibility for my learning and what I could contribute to the unit and my patients' well-being.
You do the same, okay?

I repeated the process above until I had a read on the crash cart stuff no matter what room I was given that shift. It really is that simple to do and will help you ease your anxiety in a way that you do not even realize until you have done it.

Setting up your Room

Nurses can be a little OCD; especially ICU nurses. We like to know where things are at, all the time. With good reason, our patients' condition can change in a second and there is generally not time to waste hunting for needed equipment.

That being said, honestly, I know this to be true on every single floor; regardless of the type of nurse you become. Floor nurses and OB nurse are not immune to patients crashing. Oncology? Forget about it, of course your patients are unstable. That's why taking some time here is essential to allaying some of your own anxiety aka fear.

We do an in-room shift change report with the off going nurse on my unit. This is not the most ideal time to assess the things that are in your room when you first start out because you will need to be paying total attention to the nurse giving you report.

Pretty quickly after that time spent with your peer learning about your patient you should be assessing your room for needed items.

Pick a spot and work around the room. Pick the same spot to start every room you assess this way Ask these kinds of questions:

What drips are going? Is the rate the same as the one on the MAR? Is there a sterile way to cap the end of any IV you need to move? Do you have labels on lines? Do you have alcohol swabs close by? Are any of the meds hangings or their tubing about to expire or be empty? Gloves need stocking up? Is there a nasal canula present if the patient is not already on oxygen? What about at least one suction setup including a younker? Is there an ambu bag that is appropriate for your patient and the correct adapter from the wall to the O2 line? We call this a Christmas tree because that is what it looks like. You have a stepstool around? Do you know how to get the bed in CPR mode quick? Is your patient on a ventilator or BiPAP? Do those machines in your hospital require switching settings in order to bleed O2 through the machine when in ambu bag mode?

You need these items on the ready even for a seemingly 'well' patient that may be about to discharge. Remember, as long as they are in your care you need to be ready for them to become unstable. They are in the hospital not the Hilton, after all. The human body can and will do crazy things and the wheels coming off is something you must be prepared for at all times.

I have heard stories of people being in a wheelchair ready to discharge that coded while paperwork was being signed. I have also been told of people with relatively minor conditions that have died waiting on resuscitation equipment. Last week a nurse was chatting with a patient ready to transfer to the floor and she suddenly lost pulse. One gal even shared that her very first patient choked on lunch and died in her presence, largely she thought, because she had no clue where to start in that situation. Since it had nothing to do with the reason for the admission she never even considered that possibility and even hitting the code button on the wall was not something she had practiced in her head.

My first personal experience with this happened in my pediatrics rotation in school. The ambu bag had been taken down the hall to a procedure room and inadvertently not returned. I replaced it and it was later needed. Luckily, my instructor had told us that very morning about the importance of safety equipment being present at all times so I checked at the start of my shift otherwise, I would not have considered it among everything else I was trying to grasp in the pediatrics rotation. I have no idea if her story was true or not. It served its purpose though.

I never wanted to be the nurse that lost a patient because I had to run to get an ambu bag or because I could not reach the person to do chest compressions. So this lesson stuck for me without having to actually live a disaster. Even after I nailed down the locations of emergency equipment and became a pro at the Pyxis I still had some uncertainty lingering around.

I figured it out by accident watching my final preceptor in my residency program. While I was busy taking report from the other nurse he was busy taking immediate control of the room. Not in a bossy pants sort of way. It was very quiet. In fact, the first few times I watched him buzz quietly around the room while I was taking report making chit chat with the patient or the family I didn't even catch it. He was looking at medication bags, checking IV lines, peeking in cupboards for linens removing unneeded equipment and the like. Then it hit me, he was assessing what he needs. He was organizing to his liking, so that in case of emergency he knew where things are located. He was removing unneeded equipment so it did not get in his way, he was looking in cupboards for linens, under pads, bath supplies and all the things he would need throughout the shift so he wasn't caught off guard and removing the bazillion syringes and filter needles that cluttered up the computer workstation space and trash that was over-flowing. He was claiming his space. Cool, huh? He was laying a firm foundation for a shift with less anxiety and more control.

I liked how he rolled. I could see how calm he was and I wanted to possess that calm. So, I copied him and you know what? It worked!

Within 2 days of claiming my space and setting up for the shift I felt so damn empowered. This was MY room and that left me feeling much more collected and ready to handle crazy things knowing that I did not have to worry that I didn't know where things were at in the room or that the trash cans were full to overflowing.

Do not underestimate the power in this simple act of claiming the space you work in for the shift. Even if the only thing you do is walk into the space and mentally say, 'I am here now + am taking excellent care of this patient'. The intent of it shifts the energy in your favor by putting you in charge of your room from word go. Let's recap how you can feel more comfy straight away.

Keep Patients Alive by Knowing these Five:

1. Where's the code blue button on the wall
2. Where's the CPR button on the bed + the stool to stand on
3. Where's the Crash cart on the floor
4. Where's the Oxygen Valve on the wall
5. Where's the Bag Mask with oxygen tubing

You may only need to ask yourself these questions 50 or so times the first month. Do it every day though so you can burn the answers into your memory banks. In an emergency you become surprisingly forgetful.

Here is another checklist (oh boy!)
Start of Shift Once-Over for Safety-Your Room Needs These:

- Is there oxygen tubing and a nasal canula?
- Is there a bag/mask/valve that is proper size/fit for the patient and appropriate to their circumstance?
- Is the oxygen adapter hooked up to the oxygen valve on the wall?
- Is there at least one suction setup? Is there a yankauer?
- Is there a stool? Is the call bell working?
- Is the bed working and is it in the lowest position and locked? Is your patient wearing socks if he can ambulate? Is there a bedpan or urinal nearby?

These are questions you should be asking every single time the shift changes on every single patient. Don't fall into the trap of thinking that all this 'stuff' is still there since you had the patient yesterday, people borrow stuff from rooms, ya know? Tape this list to the back of your badge. It only takes one time to be missing one of these things for a patient to be harmed. Better safe...

Focus Point: Worrying that you will forget something is a waste of your intelligence! Carry the right tools, know where to find things and claim your space each shift to tame the worry-bot and feel empowered; even as a new nurse.

Action Step: Go find the crash cart on your floor.

Mantra Mojo: *I will learn step up and claim my space quickly each shift and in doing so will be calm in the middle of the storm.*

Dear Overwhelmed Yet Amazingly Awesome Nurse-

All these lists you are making are extra work I know, but wow, they help!

You are worth any amount of work it takes to dissolve any fear you may be feeling around your new work gig.

They do not just let anyone squeak thru nursing school, you know?

You really are smart.
Let yourself be smart.
You got this on lock!
Love
Me

MENTAL PREP + ATTITUDE ADJUSTING

So, you've determined what tools you need in your pockets, awesome!

You have your room setup to your liking and you know where everything is at, right? You know where the crash cart is located and where to get things from the Pyxis in a pinch. So you are going to be *physically* prepared for something extreme to happen.

Right on, Nurse Awesome!! Way to be prepared!

Now there is a bit of mental work to be done. Cause really, what are you going to do with all that equipment in the right place at the right time if you don't know how to use it?

Nothing but stand there feeling dumb. Trust me, I have been there.

Think about the emergency situations that you and your patient could face. Aside from the obvious one, coding, why are they in the hospital?

Sometime after your initial assessment of your patient each shift, you need to spend a minute and run through the emergency situations in your head that might happen for that patient. If they have chest pain what will you do? If they experience flash pulmonary edema what will you do? What if they are having trouble breathing or if you walk into them unresponsive or they are seizing? What happens next?

I know this may seem silly to you. I know you thought that once you left nursing school you would never have to role play again. I get it. There is not a grade here. It just helps you and that patient you want to keep alive to go thru things in your brain a few times. Seriously you guys, try it.

This is one of those areas that will give you anxiety because you don't know what you don't know. Spend some time in your room looking at the setup and imagining yourself in those pinch situations. I swear this will help you.

I know, I know. It is easy to make the assumption that because you both practiced + tested on those things in school that you will transfer that knowledge to your job.

That works with some things yes, other not so much. For example, if you were like me you probably spent endless hours practicing Foley catheterization and IV starts on lab dummies, right? The first time you did this skill on a person you learned that the steps in your brain and muscle memory engrained during lab time were only small pieces.

Unfortunately not at all like the real thing.

My first actual time to catheterize a female patient in the ICU was successful, but not without the help of another nurse. My patient came from the Emergency Department actively trying to die, crashing, she was sick and there were 4 people in the room with me and tons of hub-bub going on. She had just been intubated emergently and the doc had just begun to hunt for the Internal Jugular with an ultrasound to insert a central line. A fellow nurse was hanging a second bolus of saline to bump her pressure up until we could get access for the levophed. So, the doc was waiting on ME to catheterize the patient to start his sterile procedure and the patient really needed the pressor support. The patient had some anatomical challenges that a lab dummy never presented. I was sweating like crazy and trying to absorb all that was going on with MY patient at the same time as I was trying to stay sterile while I cathed the patient.
I cannot even tell you how many times I did this skill in lab and in my OB rotation. This time, I was a klutz and it may as

well have been my first time doing this skill, ever.

Same thing with IV starts. Patients are all different. The veins on the lab dummies are plump and juicy and generally well marked by the needle sticks of your countless predecessors. You know where you are going, you can see the vein, and the blood that comes out is lab blood which doesn't scare you quite like real blood does once it gets flowing. There is not a live person on the other end of that needle to wince and jerk and freak out as you search for a vein.

Knowledge-wise you are prepared for the task but mentally, in the heat of things, it will be much different.
(Note to Self: you are *qualified just not prepared*.)

Foley's and IV's give you a little wiggle room. Blue patients do not. So, while school qualifies you, it is only your experience that prepares you. Obviously, those blue patients are something you need to be prepared for before you experience them. The first time you have an emergency or actually code one of your patients you are going to need to be prepared in a way that no lab time can possibly prepare you for, right?

Don't misunderstand me. ACLS, code days at school and all gave me a bit of comfort because I knew the basic steps I needed to take, however; it is not the same as the real deal. When I realized how little I was actually prepared now that this was my show and my show alone, I began running through things mentally at least once per shift per patient. This helped me more than I can express.

My point is that I could have sat waiting until I actually had my first emergency. For me though, the learning curve of a patient being alive or dead was just too steep. Nothing will cause your adrenaline to spin off the damn charts like a decompensating patient will. It is worth noting here that my first patient code was 6 months into my job. If I had waited I would have been nervous a long time!

What are some of those adrenaline-spinning events, you ask? Here:

What do you do for chest pain?
What do you do for low oxygen saturation?
What do you do for sudden shortness of breath?
What do you do for a seizing patient?

Those nurses that you admire have the benefit of time on their side. They have practiced a lot. They know the facility protocol well. So take a minute and practice mentally:

What do you do for chest pain?

- Note the time the pain started for them. Is the patient in for a heart issue? If so the doc has probably left some instructions.
- You are going to want to get an EKG stat. If you work on the telemetry monitored floor call the monitor tech and ask them to look at what is going on for the patient. If you monitor your own strips go look for PVC's, a run of V-tach, ST elevation or other irregular activity.
- Are they there for a respiratory issue? It might be causing the pain but since you are not a doc you will not make that call. Keep going with your interventions.
- Ask them to describe and rate the pain. Is it the worst pain they have ever felt? Is it constant or intermittent? Is it sharp and stabbing? Burning? Crushing? Worse on inspiration? Will a position change help them? Are they still in pain no matter how they are sitting?

- Are there any other symptoms like shortness of breath or diaphoresis?

If they are having that crushing type pain that does not stop better get some O2 on them, find the aspirin, nitro and morphine orders quickly and get them into your patient.

Did your intervention work?
Do they still have pain?
Did you call the admitting doc or the cardiologist for this patient?

You should!

Now be an awesome nurse and go find out what your hospital wants you to do specifically when a patient is reporting chest pain.

Do you just call the Rapid Response Team or are there some specific interventions that you need to be doing while you call the team and doctor?

** Add your facility or floor protocol here**

What do you do for low oxygen saturation?

- Locate the bag mask and oxygen equipment in the room. Wait, you already did that at shift change, right? So you are ahead of the game in this potential crisis. Yay, you!
- Determine how low is low. Is this a COPD patient that is used to low SpO2? 85% may not be so bad for them.
- Look at them. Assess them. Are they symptomatic? If the monitor says the patient has an SpO2 of 75% and the patient is talking to you and not grey/blue then this is probably not accurate.
- Check the pulse oximeter probe to make sure it is attached to the patient well. If the monitor says they are 75% and they are using accessory muscles to breathe you better get some help, now.
- Are they breathing effectively? When you look at them are they hard to arouse? Are their respirations slow? Have you given them too much narcotic or benzo? Get the reversal drugs for those and give it to them.
- Are they having trouble breathing? Get some oxygen on them and crank it up. Is it helping? Put the head of their bed as high as their condition will allow so they can expand those lungs.

Look. I need, need, need you to understand this as a new nurse.

Sometimes your patients will quit breathing properly. Said patient will not give a flying crap that you are a new nurse.

RN behind your name means some things for sure and one of that is that you know how to operate the O2 equipment, that you can manage an O2 delivery device, including a bag mask, and that you can get it on your patient when they need it.

You cannot lose your shit in this moment. You must breathe

for the patient if they are cyanotic or dusky or barely expanding their chest with each inhalation and their SPO2 reads in the low 80's.

Stay with your patient, push the code light on the wall, use the phone or holler out the door for help. Do not leave a patient that is struggling to breathe to get more help. Do something to help him in the room until more help arrives.

So this is going to be scary. The adrenaline surge is crazy. First because it is usually an unexpected thing and second because there is literally someone's life in your hands at that moment. The heaviness of that will smack you in the face.

You are going to help yourself by running a 'holyshitmyguystoppedbreathing' moment each time you go into your patients' room for the first time in shift. Every shift.

Walk thru the things you would do in this scenario. Where is the O2? Is it ready to go? Is there at least a nasal canula in your room? Is there an ambu bag? How would you get the Rapid Response Team + your charge nurse?

After a dozen or so shifts this will become habit, which means you will be able to take some action instead of freaking out and standing still in the moment of crisis. Got it, Nurse Awesome? Now find out your facility specific rules and list them here:

What do you do for sudden shortness of breath?

- Assess the situation. Are they involved in an activity or sitting in bed? Are they also tachycardic with the shortness of breath? Is their SpO2 low too?
- Do the easy things first. If all the vitals look good and the patients pallor has not changed then reassure them that they are getting enough oxygen. See if you can work your magic and get them to relax. Maybe this is just a bit of anxiety or they just overdid that walk around the floor.
- Sit the head of their bed up as high as their condition allows.
- Listen to their lung sounds. Do they sound clear or are they sounding a bit like a clothes washer? If you hear wetness you need to put some oxygen on the patient or turn it up if already on them, call the RT team who may change the method of delivery of said oxygen and then call the doctor. Maybe they are having some pulmonary edema. If you hear no breath sounds in one of the fields you should do the same; it might be a pneumothorax. Don't forget to look at their trachea; tension pneumo can kill a patient quickly. Are they stridoris? Do they have respiratory issues in their history?

Knowledge is power, phenoms.

Empower yourself a bit more by listing out your facility specific instructions here.

What do you do for a seizing patient?

- If you start your shift with a patient that has a history of seizure then please have these bulleted items in your head straight away. Do not wait for a seizure to happen, k?
- Keeping your patient safe is your first priority, yes? Let someone know if your patient starts seizing. That may be a doc on duty or the charge nurse; it depends on your facility.
- Make sure you have a suction set up in the room with a yankauer. Make sure that you have oxygen setup if the patient is not on it already.
- Make sure that you know the difference in seizures, not all seizures are grand mal. Do not try to suction them while they are seizing, this is for the postictal stage.
- Don't' forget to pad the rails + keep the bed in the lowest position Make sure suction and oxygen is readily available. Keep environmental stimulus down to a minimum.
- If they are seizing it is going to scare you the first time. Don't panic. It is hard to watch, they may turn blue, make noises, lose continence. There O2 sat may drop rapidly as they hold their breath and such. Their vitals will most likely go nutso. If family is in the room you will need to reassure them, too.
- It is important to note the time it started and the type of movement you see. The doctor will ask you about it so pay attention. Do their eyes deviate to one side? Are the movements big and bilateral to upper and lower extremities or focused in one area only? Are they rhythmic or jerky? What happened prior to that event?
- Try to get them on their side as much as possible, their head in particular so you they do not aspirate anything. Make sure their airway is not obstructed but do NOT put anything in their mouth, please.
- Holler for some Ativan; if they do not come out of it

within a minute you will need to give them some. (Look at your PRN drugs at the start of your shift if you have a patient on seizure precaution. Is there an order for Ativan on the PRN list? If not, call a doctor and get one now instead of waiting until they seize.

- The doc will mostly ask you draw labs to check levels of their anti-seizure medication. So be prepared for this too.

Once they stop seizing they will most likely be confused. Plan to spend a bit of extra time with them to reorient and reassure them.

Again, take a minute and ask your fellow nurses what Smiley General wants you to do if your patient has a seizure.

Add your facility or floor protocol here

Attitude Adjustments

While you are busy checking your room setup and running through 'worst-case scenarios' in your head there is one more thing you need to make sure you check frequently throughout your shift:

Your attitude.

Yep, YOU, Nurse Awesome, check your attitude or what I call

'taking my own temp'. Check it often for best results and

make adjustments accordingly. How are you feeling?
Are you smiling at your co-workers and patients? Are you feeling overwhelmed and freaked out? Are you pissed off at the call bell ringing over and over?

Busy days can leave you so honed in on what is going on in your immediate surroundings that you have no time to look around you. They can leave you feeling a little cranky.

A string of busy days when you feel like you are drowning in tasks can leave you feeling like you seriously hate your new job. I don't want you to underestimate how important your state-of mind is during your transition to your new nursing gig.
It can make or break you, seriously.

You have to let go of things that go wrong.

You have to take your breaks.

You have to nourish yourself.

You have to stop expecting perfection from yourself.

You have to find someone that you can talk things out with in a productive manner instead of just complaining about being overwhelmed or stuffing it inside you.

Focus Point: You have to figure out how to know when your cup is 'full' and then take the steps to empty it.

Action Step: Go get a massage or go to a movie. Take some action that says you are loving yourself up when you feel 'off'. This is just as essential as learning where that crash cart is located on your floor.

Mantra Mojo: *I will stay fully present in this moment and remain open to all good things coming this shift*

Enough about your attitude; you get it, I know.

Let's look at what happens in your world all day.

COURSE CORRECTIONS

While we are in the whole mental attitude space I wanted to share a few more things with you.

These are some of the more powerful thoughts that helped me shift my focus quickly + stay in an open head-space.

The way to course correct when my shit got jacked, yo!

> *First, Don't waste time with anger at your school for not teaching you 'all this' or not preparing you. Anger will not change it + there is so much to learn you'd of been in school forever trying to learn it. Be thankful they helped you pass the NCLEX; this was the focus of their job.

> *Celebrate everything! Getting that name RN badge, remembering to document, communications breakthroughs with a patient, being on time with your medications, I mean everything! These may seem small however; in these first months of your career they are HUGE. You must pat yourself on the back as your awesomeness happens. Dance in the supply closet if you need to, just celebrate your success!

> Positive in=positive out.

> *Set an intention before the shift. Hold a picture in your mind of the kind of shift you want. Set intention before you enter the patient's room for the first time. Focusing your energy on the best outcome for both of y'all holds healing power. You typically get what you expect to get.

*You will be seriously stressed out if you focus on what you *need* to learn. Shift that focus instead to what you **do** know and practice it. Focusing on things you're good at will build your confidence. Plus, the other stuff only comes with time so no sense fussin over it now.

*Speak up if you are asked to do a procedure that you know nothing about. No one wants you to hurt a patient, break sterile field, or whatever. Most folks will help you along here; if not they will ask for someone with more experience. Do not get your feelings hurt by this-it is purely professional. Take notes and learn so that next time you can help out.

*Speaking of feelings, learn how to not take things personally and you will spare yourself a lot of heartache. Things are rarely ever personal and when they are, most medical professionals will not hesitate to tell you they are.

*Spend some time quietly with yourself each day so you can know what 'peaceful' feels like to you. This will help you I.D. the opposite, which of course, is stress. You will need to know what it feels like for you so you can stop it before you reach that overwhelmed + meltdown point.

*Stuff the absolute must-do nursing interventions for different conditions common to your area of specialty in your head or on note cards in your pockets so that you can use it if needed in pinch. You still need to be able to save a life while learning.

*Don't be afraid to ask questions but try to choose the correct time to ask questions. For example, the middle of a code is not the time to ask why Sodium Bicarbonate is beneficial to a coding patient.

*Be proactive. Look things up yourself. Go ask your peers questions with at least some information on the subject already.

*Be the person that volunteers to do everything. Foley, IV, rectal tube: the more you can get your hands on things the quicker your experience and confidence will grow.

*Do not let anything get you down for long. Shake off the tough stuff and do not wallow in your mistakes.
At least once a shift these first few months you will feel like you want to quit. Hang tough there, superstar!

You will make it!

You can't really make all the feelings of newness and uncertainty go away when you first start caring for patients on your own.

Taking some time and being prepared, finding out what your hospital wants from you, learning the equipment and adjusting your own attitude each day will go a long way towards removing the jitters you feel.

Take a breath and add the steps above to your practice so you feel a little more in control and a lot more peaceful as you learn the ropes of new-nurse-dom.

Dear Nurse Awesome, Your license does not read Crankypants, RN. You have to figure out how to let the stupid stuff that happens each shift go. It is really doing you no good to hold onto it. There is not one person benefiting from your grumpiness. Especially not you so do what you need to change this for yourself.

Dance Yoga Ice Cream Whatever! Love-Your better happier half-M

A DAY IN THE LIFE

So how are you feeling about the day-to-day responsibilities of your new career? Have you gotten a good handle on what is expected of you yet? Ask as many questions as it takes until you feel good and cozy with your boundaries when it comes to patient care, the choices you are empowered to make on your floor and those that you need to clear through a doc or your charge nurse. Your preceptor should be able to help draw some clear lines for you so you can feel capable of decision-making within those lines from day one of your job.

I entered my job believing I had a strong handle on what a typical day would look like for me. I had practiced in my school clinical time for 2 years, after all.. The last few months of school I was actually doing my clinical days on the unit I went to work in, so there were no questions and little fear wrapped around the actual day-to-day responsibilities of a nurse on this unit for me.

ZERO, I tell you. None!

Surprise! This was the largest area of adjustment for me personally. There was not one thing typical about the day and it was not much like my clinical experience.

I had zero idea what nurses *really* do all day.

The fact that I just spent 2 years of clinical in a fancy-pants nursing program left me a tad pissy about this whole deal. I was exposed to enough clinical days that I felt I should have seen this coming. All the pieces were there; they just weren't put together in a cohesive way. Not even in that last semester when I was supposed to be doing 'real' nursing.

If you don't understand this yet please note that as a nurse you will be expected to function much like the hub of a wheel. You will be the controller of all the movement and action with the patient.

You do NOT do that in school. Even when you are supposed to be doing that your school preceptor will not give over the reins totally. It is a problem.

In addition to the giving medications on-time and correctly there was the patient care to be done. Hygiene, grooming and meals, you know all that caring for the patient stuff.

Then there was patient education which is an important part of what we do daily. Chatting with patients+ their families about the new disease process they will be taking home with them is not for sissies. You might feel a little pressure knowing that you are responsible for teaching them about the care and feeding that their illness that will surely demand of them. It can be overwhelming to know that you're the one providing the tools they need to take control of it in a way that empowers them rather than totally debilitating them. Furthermore, there is no one that will have your back and fill in blanks you missed like when you were a student. Yes, you will have a preceptor for a bit, they may or may not pay much attention to this area since it is just a small piece of the day.

Getting used to being on your own with just those pieces to address is enough to throw you into stress response.

Add to that, chatting with doctors from various disciplines about my shift assessment, asking for various changes to the medications or restrictions placed on the patient based on that assessment, issues with pain management for that patient, transporting patients to new rooms, to scans and procedures, counseling services ranging from grief response to positive thinking and just about every topic in between, assisting with death planning, explaining procedures, deciphering medical jargon, post-mortem care, drawing labs, cleaning rooms and taking out trash, coordinating care between disciplines, working with social work to help with deficiencies in insurance, home health assistance and the like, ordering lunch for a patient, being the peacemaker in a crazy family dynamic, painting a clear yet compassionate picture with the jumbled up realities the doc left behind, correcting Dr. Google....I did very little of this in school.

These are all just the 'expected' job functions that come with that RN title of yours and they are the invisible piece of ninja skill you cannot be taught.

You get the picture, right?

I really only had a tiny clue as to what I was walking into as 'the nurse'. The feeling of overwhelm became my new reality as I learned to sort out my role in the patients stay.

As the person in the middle of all this you kind of need to know a little about all of this, right?

By the end of my first month I had a good handle on the 'unwritten' job assignment that nursing school never mentioned.

The hard part was not so much the tasks themselves but the fact that you never knew when they would come at you. Sure, you could sort of predict that unit rounds would happen before 10 but exactly when was a crap shoot. The various consults with PT, ST, and Dietary you can never predict. When the specialists rounded was not even worth a guess.

It can make for a chaotic day.

Equally shocking, I felt like I was constantly in a hurry. I never had enough time for anything. And dang it, as a brandy-newy nurse I needed time to look up drug interactions, to complete tasks that experienced nurses do in a flash, to figure out how to put all the pieces together into a picture that made sense.

Time I did not have.

So remember in school how exciting it was for you to know that your patient needed a Foley or a new IV line? Remember how you would take 30 minutes just to prepare and go over the procedure in your head before you even tried? This resembles the real-world of daily RN life exactly 0%, none at all.

In the real world you do not get an unlimited amount of time to review procedure in your head or book.

You do not get to stop and regroup and you do not get to default to your primary nurse when things get tough cause, duh, you ARE the primary nurse. You are now the primary nurse and that takes some getting used to; even though it is a happy kind of thing.

So the general answer to the question, 'What will I be doing all day?' is 'providing patient care' the detailed view of that could take an entire day just to explain to someone not in nursing.

The first time I told my husband about a patient that I ordered lunch for that was ticked cause he got orange and not strawberry sorbet my husband looked at me like what I was telling him did not compute. He said, uhm, why are you ordering lunch, you didn't go to school to be a waitress.

Truth. Nor a hostess at the Hilton, or project manager

or day planner, but you will be all of these things

I don't want you to have to struggle with the stress for long. It changes the way you process information and can harm the way you nurse your patients. Not to mention it makes you crankypants.

I found these things helped me get out of the weeds quickly, try them and see if they help you, Nurse Awesome:

- ✓ Plan as much as you can but expect changes: if you get so locked into things occurring in a certain order it will make you nuts when things get changed
- ✓ Get in front of things when you have down time. For example, if you are open for an admission and you know that your other 3 patients need certain things that must be done in the day but they are not time-sensitive things then do them early in the shift. Before you get hit with an admission and all the extra work that comes with them
- ✓ Organize yourself and use some of those awesome prioritization skills school taught
- ✓ Use a brain sheet: This just helps you keep your patient data in one place. It is a life-saver
- ✓ Chart as you go: Develop the habit of charting real-time and you will not have to play catch-up. You do not get to leave things uncharted like you did when you were a student
- ✓ Stay away from cliques: Mind your business and don't gossip. It wastes time.
- ✓ Learn how to laugh at yourself, some days it is all that saves your brain from implosion; one of my favorite sayings during my transition to the ICU.."some days you're the windshield, some days you're the bug"
- ✓ Work smart first, hard second: This means that you use your skills to organize and prioritize before you get started with your day not 3 hours into it.

- ✓ Look at how the experienced nurses around you handle themselves: I cannot stress enough how important it is to watch the masters in action before you try to reinvent the wheel.
- ✓ Accept that this will probably make you nuts the first few months: You will want to be faster than you are, cut yourself some slack. You will stay late. I have friends that were miserable for 6 months until one day things just clicked. Now they are at home one their floor and in their new role as R.N. and they never stay late to work to catch up.

It is a challenge this first month to learn the flow of all this activity. Once you get the hang of it you will be amazed at how well you juggle multiple and competing priorities'.

Try to show yourself a little extra TLC while you get adjusted and please do not expect that you will have the flow of your day under control within the first 30 days.

It takes a while before you start to feel like you are running the days instead of the other way around.

Focus Point: Prepare yourself to be flexible while you are learning the flow of the day on your floor. It will keep you from going nuts.

Action Step: Let go of the need to have everything go exactly the way that you planned it. Things get messed up and there is nothing you can do about it.

Mantra Mojo: *I will remain calm, cool and open to all possibilities that come my way this shift because I am a confident and capable RN.*

Take 5...

5 essential skills you didn't practice during school simulation lab

Juggling opposite tasks Delivering bad news Decoding doctor language Delaying gratification+ ordering chaos Seeing the big picture when there is not clear evidence to support

5 causes to champion

Advanced Directives + Living Wills
Exercise + weight contro
l Stress relief Moderation in drinking
Finding a source of joy in your life

5 things that surprise you in the first 30 days

School is just the beginning of the learning process Your peers treat you as equal the minute you tag RN on your badge You will be more tired yet more fulfilled than ever People think RN=MD. Expect to be asked to diagnose medical issues Kindness + compassion are sometime the only things that matter

DEAR NURSE AWESOME

YOU DIDN'T KNOW YOU WOULD BE THE
CENTER OF IT ALL, DID YA?

WHILE YOU ARE PLANNING TO TAKE CARE
OF THE WORLD VIA ONE PATIENT AT A
TIME DON'T FORGET TO TAKE EXCELLENT
CARE OF YOU.

WHAT ARE YOU DOING TO MAKE YOUR OWN
HEALTH PRIORITY IN THE MIDDLE OF THIS
NEW CAREER?

FIND SOMETHING⋯

LOVE YOU TONS, WANT YOU HEALTHY

ME

SHIFT REPORT

I am certain that you spent some time in school both taking and giving shift report to other nurses.

How do you feel about it now that you are in 'big leagues'? Are you nervous? Try not to be, you get the hang of this quickly.

This is one of the areas that made me super nervous as a student but that for some odd reason I believed would magically become easy when I became a nurse. I was obsessed with the thought of forgetting something important when I was a student so I left many shifts worried I had left off some piece of data that might cause my patient harm.

In school, I was much more comfortable taking report than I was giving one to another nurse because I knew most of the questions to ask and I had my handy-dandy report sheet to help me get organized. It was giving information that caused my stumble.

You will notice quickly that each nurse does their own 'thing' when it comes to report. Yes, we are all supposed to follow a guideline so you get the basics. It is just that everyone has a different area they get obsessive over while in report. I have noticed that there is typically a past incident that caused the nurse problems that is tied to that 'thing' they always want to know in more detail than you can provide.

On my unit the report used to make me nuts. I was trying so hard to give the right report that I felt totally twisted around with everyone wanting different information. One nurse wanted to know when blood sugar checks were due while another focused on lab values like BUN/Creatinine levels, while yet another was only concerned about when you gave the last dose of Ativan. Hard to get a flow going when everyone is different.

People have odd quirks. Try not to gripe about them because none of that will change them. The truth is that you have some quirky report issues too, you just don't see them is all. Just laugh off the nurse that wants to go through every detail not remotely related to that patients visit and go ahead and help the nurse that needs you to turn the patient with them before you leave.
I just had to let go of the need for a cookie-cutter approach when it came to report time. Then my stress level went down to something manageable.

There was this other thing for me, too. As ridiculous as it sounds, there was a big part of me hung up on the notion that the nurses I was giving report to were laughing at me silently in their head as I gave report.

As an older student with a professional background, the notion of being laughed at was a bit of a blow for my ego to take. I could logically conclude that with all their years of experience they had every right to be silently judging the quality of the data I was giving them at shift change, but laughing, I could not stomach. After all, as a student nurse there was no way I would always be able to decipher the important facts to communicate as a nurse that should be second nature and that excuse was no longer an option.

Anyway, age + experience aside, without an abundance of positive reinforcements for your newly acquired report-giving skills, or the time to stop and ask them to rate your performance so that you could improve things it is hard to know you are getting better and easy to feel your are the butt of all jokes. Without a trusty grade sheet like in school there was no formal measure that I could turn to in order to know I was improving either.

Frustrating when you come from the land of constant grading, to step into the real-world with no measure at all, freaked me out more than I anticipated. Making it worse for me personally, I thought the R.N. on my badge would silence my wonky feelings around shift report so I didn't really take any action in school to correct it. I was wrong; I just felt more pressure to know exactly what information to give and collect and truly expected to be able to do it quick and concise from word go.

I didn't really expect that reaction from myself. I thought that ditching school would also get rid of some of that self-imposed pressure. Not true, I was actually still expecting myself to be perfect within this new peer group. I am not sure what your expectations of yourself are at this point. I hope this chapter softens them.

Remember, perfection is not realistic! This is your practice not your perfect!

You can take at least *some* pressure off yourself here by utilizing SBAR and the Review of Systems Model to guide the flow of data you provide. Start at the top and work your way down.

No one likes to jump all over the place so try to be organized. Did you use SBAR in school? We were asked to but there was no formal enforcement so I needed some additional practice. If you were like me it would serve you well to practice it. Do everything in your life in SBAR until you get the hang of it.

Create your grocery list from it, talk to your kids about doing their chores with it, talk on the phone using it. Seriously, the more you practice the less you have to think about it at shift change and that is a good thing.

Most helpful if you find yourself with a stutter-step here? Just ask yourself what you want someone to tell you and then share that information. Sharing is caring, people.

These will help too: Is there a lab trough that is due before the next dose of that medicine which happens to be due at 0800? Tell them that in report cause chances are they will be running around hanging meds and not see the order for trough until that antibiotic is given at 0800.

Is there a test coming up first thing in the morning that needs some prep work from the nurse? Share it, please.

Is there a lab value that you reported as critical or that you had to take action on? Don't forget to pass that on.

Is there an important order about to expire? Let them know.

Is there a dietary restriction or allergy that needs to be considered? Say something about it.

Is there a psychosocial issue that needs to be kept in mind when dealing with the family? Like say, a new diagnosis of a devastating disease or difficulty thinking of at home care? You will make friends if you do not let the new nurse find out this tidbit about her daily charge on her own.

Don't forget, there will be a ton of acronyms thrown at you. If you do not know them stop and ask that nurse to explain. If they use PE to describe Pulmonary Embolism and you think that PE means Pleural Effusion or Pedal Edema well, this can make the difference in the care you provide. Better clarify and ruffle the nurses' feathers than assume and harm your patient. Clarify your abbreviations and acronyms. Don't speak in acronyms unless you both know what in the king hell you are talking about, please.

If you had to comb through the notes to find something then you can bet the other nurse will as well. If it is important for the nurse to know from the start of shift then please, tell them so they do not have to dig.

Another way to fit in faster on your floor? Be prepared when you come onto the floor. That nurse is ready to go home after a 12 hour shift; she does not want to play. It will be worse if you get report from several different nurses and your patients are strung from one end of the unit to the other. Get your butt to work on time and gather paper, pens and stethoscopes before you approach the off-going nurse.

You will gain the respect of your new peer groups more quickly if you are considerate. Nothing sucks like waiting 5 minutes for the nurse coming on shift to 'get her stuff together'. 5 minutes feels like forever, especially when you have been hard at it for 12 hours and know you have to come back that night.

While building trust with your new peer group is important, bear in mind that at the end of the day it is not the responsibility of the nurse leaving shift to give you lab values and this 'other' information that is hidden in the chart. It's your job to check for the variables.

It is nice to think that everyone will be kind to you and leave some breadcrumbs on the trail however; it is a better to cultivate the habit of leaning on yourself early in your career.

You worked hard to get here, it is now your license to protect, so do it.

You can eat up a lot of bandwidth worrying about the quality of your report but there are much wiser uses for your energy in the first month wearing your shiny new RN kicks.

It helped settle me down to remember that report style was just about as individual as our fingerprints; not everyone's is the same and they do not need to be in order to be useful. Some nurses wanted a lot of detail and others just the high points. Some feverishly wrote down every word I said while others barely glanced in my direction as they listened to what I had to share about the patient while still some others went along without writing down a single thing. The people who write down nothing are especially intimidating. You are talking and they are just staring at you, nodding there head but noting nothing at all. This will make you feel like your report sucks, most likely though that they are taking careful notes in their head and do not need to jot stuff down. Yes, believe it or not, there are nurses out there with these kinds of memory skills.

Just keep steady ahead giving report. What they do with it is up to them, not you.
(Note to Self: Don't try to adjust your style based on someone else's.)

Just do your thing and do it well and that will be plenty enough here. If you still find yourself a bit nervous just pretend you are giving report to yourself and share everything from that chart that you would want to know. If they don't need the data they do not have to use it but at least you provided it so you can leave shift with a clear conscience.

When all else goes sideways gather + give this information

as the rock bottom need-to-knows:

- Allergies+ Code Status
- Admission date and admission diagnosis
- Neurological status
- Diet + Activity orders
- Blood glucose check times +Any med that is due soon
- Any PRN they have given recently

This will keep people from hating you.

What are you going to do with all the data you gather during shift report anyway? Let's find out!

Focus Point: Be one time and give a clear, concise report.

Action Step: Notice how other nurses give you report. Are there items being given to you that you are not giving to other nurses? Observing is the best teacher when it comes to upping the quality of your report skills quickly.

Mantra Mojo: *I will not devalue myself or my work by comparing myself to more experienced nurses.*

Hey There Nurse Phenom–

Find something in each day to feel good about. Replay that 'good' thing in your head as you walk to your car each day after your shift.

Even your small victories should be celebrated.

Believe it or not managing to get a demented patient off a bedpan without spilling pee everywhere is a victory! It may not seem like much if you have never been in that situation before, right?

Even this seemingly small thing IS a victory!

Think Like a Nurse in the Real World

You knew this day would come, right?

Here is your reward for those years of study and sacrifice.

Time to be a nurse!

You got a great hand-off report at shift change. You have met your patients and done the quick safety checks of the room. You are prepared for an emergency.

Now the day can begin.

Since each of your patients is different, the day will look different for each of them, right? Despite the different activities you must plan you are the one that gets to plan most of them; not just the nursing ones. Bet you didn't realize that in school, huh?

As the nurse you are like Mission Control for your patients' day.

The Big Kahuna, Kingpin, Boss-Man, 'The Don' of everything that has anything to do with this patient in your care for 12 hours.

I emphasize this because it is important that right away you know that you need to coordinate it all. I failed to realize this during my first months on deck and because of t hat things were more dicey than they needed to be for me. I deferred to other nurses and specialities as to what my patient 'should or should not' be doing and when exactly each thing would happen in the day. I ran myself ragged by allowing everyone but me to run the show.

Remember, you are not just a nurse you are THE nurse.

I was so unorganized that I was constantly backtracking and referring to my brain sheet to keep patients straight. It was highly inefficient but I had to go through it to figure out how to stop doing it.

When I stepped into my role fully and proclaimed myself the Big Kahuna (in my mind not out loud) for all my patients the inefficient energy in my shifts turned quickly to my favor. Best I can figure, the hub of the wheel aspect of job is one of the primary reasons for all that emphasis on critical thinking in school not to mention all that pressure that felt needless as we moved through skills lab testing and clinical.

It might even be the reason they leave you floundering for answers in theory when we ask them to teach us to 'think like a nurse'. You know, so that when you get your first job as a nurse you will land on your feet when you are thrown in head first and become 'the Don'. *(**Note to Self:** Forgive your instructors)*

Make sense?

So, what they do not tell you in school is that critical thinking is just a fancy way to say this…

Combine what you learned about the body and disease in theory class with what you learned about patient care with what you learned about pharmacology + psychology to all the facts about the patient that is in front of you at each moment in time to plan and conduct care based on all of that data and then draw conclusions in order to make more decisions for that patient.

So here is the scene. You walk into work at 630am+ you have no idea what type of patients you will be taking care of that day. Unlike nursing school these folks are just sprung on you and they are different every single day. Today you have a mixed bag. Your patients include a 50 yr old with COPD, a 20 year old amputee that had muscle flap procedure done to correct a pressure ulcer, a 30 year old post gallbladder that woke up slow from anesthesia so the doc admitted them for observation, and an 80 year old with new onset a-fib and dementia.

Each of them has tests to be done today, labs to be looked at, medicines to give, and PT orders to consider. Don't forget about all the psychosocial implications of their illness. Oh yea, they also need to eat and toilet today, at least once. There is a lot to get done and without someone actually feeding you each step to take and then waiting for you to take it like in school, this can get hard and overwhelming and leave you feeling much less than awesome.
Here is where you get to apply your theory chops and think like a nurse in a real world to make a difference in the life of your patient.

Just hearing report on your patients should already have your mind turning through care plan and disease process data to get an idea of what your day will look like, right? Of course, you learned about these disease states in school. You have made dozens of care plans with these types of patients so don't panic. You got this thing on lock! Just walk through it one step at a time.

COPD you should think about breathing, right? A young amputee will probably be a full dose of pain, some infection prevention and psych issues. The chole will need some pain control and diet teaching and you will need to monitor your fibber for hemodynamic stability and symptoms of poor perfusion and be worried about coagulation issues.

Amazingly, you do not need to have 3 medical nursing diagnosis statements and a few psych statements with multiple goals +interventions like you did in school.

Focus on just the top stuff, sweets!

I know you've determined as shift report went along which person you would see first, right? If not, start to train your brain to shift into nurse mode before report is even done.

Peek on each of your patients. Are they alive and breathing? Great focused assessment skills! Now what is next?

Diagnose what you see as your biggest issues this day on the way to grab the first round of meds for the shift.
Plan what you need to do while you are standing at the Pyxis and implement your plan as you give that first medication pass of the day.

It does not have to be like the huge and elaborate plan that you created to please your professors. Maybe you plan to help your COPD patient with hygiene that day so they oxygenate efficiently, using the time to assess and teach.

Maybe you chat with the young amputee to get a feel for how they are adjusted psychosocially and teach them about diabetes control while you are helping them order breakfast.

Next medication pass at noon, maybe when trays go out at lunch assess the steps you took. How is your patient doing? What has changed? What do you need to do based off of what is different?

Use the same nursing process steps when you do your chart review on each patient.

What is the H&P assessment data from the physician saying is the overall plan? How will your care support the docs? Are all the orders that need to get written to make the plan happen get completed?

Have you done what the doc asked to be done? Is there something you need to add to their labs for the day? Do you need to remove a Foley, start a new IV or change a dressing?

Look at the test results and apply the nursing process. ADPIE, remember?

Combine that with a little prioritization with the help of Monsieur Maslow. Who gets seen first and why?

Reassess as you give meds, compare the plan you had against the plan you have now. Make adjustments.

Lather. Rinse. Repeat. All day.
Using the nursing process should be so routine for you by now that you do it without even realizing you are doing it.

Seriously, if you plan your day using the nursing process, especially the first year on the job, then you will not miss important aspects of the patients care.

It will keep you from making a knee-jerk choice about patient care. It will force you or guide you through a logical thinking pathway. Always assess first, always evaluate what you did before you change direction and do something different. Always use evidence-based practice in the care you provide.

That said there are some situations when you need to just act quickly; you know the ones. So, just like the professor said a million times, be flexible and adjust your actions when needed.

I spoke to several of the nurses around me that I could see knew their stuff. They are rarely in a panic mode, always time to visit with patient and guide families through decision-making, mostly happy nurses.

I asked them how they survived the first 6 months. Some of them said therapy, others said whiskey, but all of them said they used some form of the nursing process every single day to guide and plan patient care.

All of them said they kept notes the first 6 months on everything they did so they could repeat it next time alone and invariably they created an individual report sheet that fit them instead of using a canned report sheet created by someone else. This is stuff that you encounter that is important to you so don't expect your list to look like your buddies. Chances are you will need some focus on things they don't need to focus on and vice-versa.
Since I wanted to be a happy nurse I followed their lead.

Focus Point: Consider all the facts and variables before you make a decision about patient care.

Action Step: Use ADPIE as much as you can this week at work. This way of thinking that you learned in school is a sure fire way to train your brain to critically think.

Mantra Mojo: *I am a confident and capable nurse who brings together many pieces of info on my patients into a workable plan with ease.*

YOUR BIBLE + YOUR BRAINS

I followed the advice of those experienced nurses that surrounded me. I took notes every day, even when I was exhausted.

Get in this habit. Jot down what you did so that you can later reflect on it; get help with it, Google it, whatever...

You will learn something and stretch yourself, every single day. When it comes to big things take some detailed notes. It will serve you well in the long run. In my own notes there was the actual procedure then there was my 'Notes to Self' scribbled in the margins, mine were something like this:

Post-Mortem Care: Determine if this is an ME case first. Call organ procurement and eye people. Get the funeral home info from the family before they leave. Make sure there are no valuables on the person. Close their eyes and mouth before rigor sets in. Change any soiled linens before family comes in.*(NTS*: removal of central lines from dead people may cause bleeding; and a lot of it (no more resistance/tone in the circulatory system.))

Some of the other NTS's in my margins:

> NTS: You will need meds to address seizures, pain, anxiety, high BP, Low BP-fast-so make sure you know what PRN meds you have at shift start.

> NTS: 7up in an NG tube clears a clogged line. Try before you pull it + use diet on diabetics.

> NTS: Tube Feed Poop is runny. If your patient has been on them without a BM then expect one and be prepared by fixing the under pad accordingly.

Others I wrote more extensive tips about...like this one on

Tube Feed Tips:
> If you will remove the old lines from the pump but leave connected to patient, then hang and prime the new bag it will be easier and less messy to put the newly primed tube feed into the patients NG tube. Use a 60 cc syringe instead of the tube feed piston that comes with the kit. The syringe is easier to push and fits in your small hand better.
>
> To clear line of gunk, especially if there is a lot of line and you have suction turned on the wall just turn stopcock off to patient then take off the orange cap on the open med/flush port, this creates suction that will pull the stuff in the tube through. You could turn off to patient and flush with water too. In a pinch take that NG that will not flush and use some diet 7-up and let it sit in a line/piston connected before you give up on it and insert a new one.

It is a lot like school; only this is where you will see things that make you go, 'Wait, uh, we didn't learn it that way in school.' Don't worry sweetness; the first 30 days will show you a lot that school could not show you and you will learn quickly what you can use and what you want to leave alone.

I cannot stress the difference it will make in both your learning and your confidence level if you will keep a notebook in your pocket or open at the desk you sit at all the time. It doesn't have to be elaborate; you just need a way to capture data. In this case the data you want to grab is any and all of the tips other nurses give you, disease process you didn't recall or need to bone up on, drug side-effects or interactions, how experienced nurses handle tough situations. It is too hard to go back at shift end and remember. The shift goes by in a blur most days this first year. I got to the point in ICU that I carried a note card in my scrub top because I didn't even have time to sit down and write things down. I knew the things I was witnessing were out-and-out nuggets of gold. I wanted them in my brain! I still carry a note card with me.

Speaking of, when it comes to your brain sheet it is good to try to use the same method you were using in school. It is good to have SOME familiarity when you enter this new world of you new job. Unless you are moving to a specialty unit and need some specifics like Station and Fundus and all that jazz, try to keep using what you are used to using.

I switched to one that was widely used on my unit. It had areas for lines and drains and drip and tubes that we see in ICU. I moved from that after a couple of months to one that I created because I don't feel I need the time slots marked out for the medications.

There are so many excellent examples of nursing brains on the web. You might want to make a mash up of several until you get one that is perfect for you. Even the best shift report and the best organizational brain sheet are no substitute for some time in the chart. Plan to be in the chart sooner rather than later, nothing screws up your day or your confidence like missing an important piece of data.

Writing notes on procedures or odd situations that you resolved in a 'bible' of some sort goes a long way to calming any anxiety you may feel over not knowing your role in the procedure. Until you have done things many times they will not be habit to you. Each nurse does things 'a little' differently. Pay attention.

Focus Point: Figuring out how to capture the flow of thinking in your own brain and creating your own nursing 'brain' or patient data sheet will also help alleviate your stress. Something about allowing your brain to work its' own way rather than like someone else's can get you in comfy spot quicker than a Xanax and a bottle of wine.

PATIENT 411

While organizing the facts on each of my patients presented little challenge for me, I was a touch freaked out with the way I come to know my patients each shift.

Remember in school how you'd spend hours combing through the chart to learn all about your patient or how the night before clinical you were immersed in textbooks to find all the care plan deets about the patient and their disease process?

I hated how staying up half the night made me so tired the day of clinical. BUT, I loved how knowing so much about my patient before I ever hit the floor made me feel so empowered.

I didn't realize how much peace of mind this provided me.

Knowing what care I was going to need to give and what skills I would utilize helped me jump around when unexpected issues came up without a freak out since I knew what to do next because of the previous nights plan.

This kind of time is a luxury not found in the real world.

Sorry, Charlie. Report comes at you hard and fast. You will be expected to have a good working knowledge of disease process and what care you need to incorporate into the day based on the patient's condition without referring to a textbook or a professor to confirm it.

Did you hear that? Without a textbook + without a professor.

Hold up there...Yes, you can do this! This is easier than you think. Your late night care plan sessions left a lot of data about patient care in your noggin. Do not doubt what you know, Nurse Awesome.

You also need to be prepared for the worst case scenario. Switching patient assignments, flexibility and continuous adjustment to your plan of care is the norm, rather than the exception like it was in school.
It helped me calm myself to come in early enough to see the chart before the shift. If you are able, plan to spend the first month getting to shift a bit early to grab your patient assignment. Seriously, do it.

Most charge nurses will have them ready 30 minutes prior to shift so it is totally doable and totally worth the extra time. Find a computer and check out important things before you get sucked up into the whirlwind of the day. Labs, meds due at shift change, procedures, the latest doctors' notes or orders that have not been released yet, PRN Meds; gather all that before report even happens.

It is truly empowering and gives you a chance to learn what you deem important for your day rather than relying on someone else to give you that data. There is nothing that feels as bad as realizing you failed to get the morning lab because you didn't notice it, especially if the off-going nurse did not mention that it is due early or that will scatter sunshine on your day like catching that disaster before it happens because you got to work a bit early.

As an aside, check with your unit about clocking in that early. Even if they will not pay you to be there early, do it for the first month; until you gain confidence. This will help both report and the beginning of your shift go so much smoother.

(Note to Self: confidence is worth more than money or sleep at this point.)

Getting out of the student mindset was not natural for me. I anticipated some issues but adjusted fairly well. You can too.

The minute you get those RN initials behind your name you are no longer in the 'student' pile and everything changes; even something as simple as giving shift report or gathering patient data. Most of the nurses you deal with will look at you as one of them. Those wonderkins that are your team mates will expect both professionalism + thoroughness from you so be prepared to give it. Drop the thought that they will be silently judging all your words and actions. Ain't no one got time for that mess like they did in school.
Be a little flexible here and don't expect every exchange to be sunshine and roses. Try as they might your co-workers will occasionally have a crummy shift so you may find yourself on the end of a bad report from time-to-time. No freaking out needed here. No matter what kind of shift report you get on a patient you can get your bearings quickly by glancing at the patients chart and snagging these essentials:

- o   Date + reason for their admission
- o   Allergy Info+Code Status
- o   Admission Diagnosis(although you may have to look in the notes to find the correct one)
- o   The latest physicians note, it will give you the plan of care
- o   Medications, PRN meds, blood sugar checks and tests due within an hour of coming on shift
- o   Labs that may need to be drawn before you give the next medication. You know troughs on antibiotics or levels on digoxin + seizure meds

The idea behind grabbing these facts before you care for the patient is to keep your patient safe and your doctors happy. Depending on your specialty you will add to or subtract from this list. Remember, knowledge is power here, Nurse Awesome.

Now, about those care plans...

WHERE HAVE ALL THE CARE PLANS GONE?

Yep, you knew it would happen, didn't you? These little darlings that you worked your tail off to master in school are absent in the real world of nursing. Remember those experienced nurses that giggled at the ream of paper you hauled into clinical each week?

Turns out they were right, you do not care plan in the real-world like you did in school. Not at all.

I was super-bummed about this at first. Was all the time I spent with research + evidenced-based care for each of your patient was just a waste?

If you are anything like me, you probably spent more time in the books creating care plans than with your family during your nursing school days.

I was shocked to find that something I spent so much time learning in nursing school was not really a large part of my actual job, at least it seemed that way my first months at Smiley General.

So, take a breath. It is not what it looks like.

It is totally true that you will never, ever, ever plan care like you did in school however; you do use all that evidence-based nursing intervention stuff you learned while creating those nursing school care plans; every single day.(**Note to Self**: no time was wasted so chill out, already.)

Technically, there is a section in every piece of charting software called 'care plans' and most hospitals ask you chart in them once a shift. So in 'some' form care plans 'do' exist.

In school I loved the process of gathering data and playing detective with my evidence but combing through the patients chart for what seemed like an eternity the night before clinical in first semester was not really my idea of a good time.

I was relieved when the marathon nights and 20 plus page reports morphed into a quick glance before shift, and a few notes jotted on scrap paper by the time we got to 4th semester.

It was cool that in the real world I would no longer be required to give up huge chunks of my life writing the same problems, goals and interventions over and over again but I expected to use at least some of that care planning prowess I had worked so hard to obtain. This was, after all, one area in which I felt I was an expert!

It was a shock when no one required me to care plan. It was weird to not have a list of goals and interventions written out to guide me or anyone to report my plan of care to in order to get approval prior to providing that care.

Check this out though, Nurse Awesome-

You are care planning + utilizing all that evidence-based stuff you learned in school. Problems, goals and interventions have not gone anywhere.

The difference is that all the work of care planning is happening in your head now instead of a piece of paper.

Seriously, in your head, Nurse Awesome!

Look at you go...

You are still performing all those nursing interventions. You just don't have an entire night before-hand to go through stacks of books to justify your care. You don't need those stacks of books now anyway. That repetition in school served you well.

You don't get to become intimately acquainted with your patient through their medical records before you ever step foot in their room however; you are so much faster now you do not need those extra hours to find what you need. (**Note to Self**: You hated those patient interviews the day before clinical anyway, remember?)

Instead, you get about 5 minutes in the room with the nurse who is leaving shift to get a report on the patient, your own physical assessment and a few minutes to look at labs and meds.

As you leave that room to go get the next patient's report you will be mentally conjuring a care plan. You can do this in your sleep.

If not, just think about these things, Nurse Awesome:

What keeps them safe?
 Where are they in Maslow's/Erikson's?
Where is their pain right now?
What is the main issue you need to address this shift?
What is an independent nursing intervention for their issues?
What is the medical reason your patient is in the hospital?
What s/s based on their medical condition would tell you that their condition is deteriorating?
What actions will you take to help them get better?
What steps will you take to support the patient while he recovers from that illness?

Short. Sweet. Easy.

Remember when you thought your instructor was crazy to give you patient after patient with the same types of issues?

Remember when you fussed because you had to learn all those lab values or when you rolled your eyes at the crazy teacher's rap song about beta blockers you were forced to learn?

Remember how you would adjust your care plans each week according to instructor feedback and still could never seem to get a care plan back from the instructor that was not covered in different colored ink corrections? If there was a game show that tested knowledge of nursing diagnoses, goals, interventions and the like we would all be the grand prize winners.

That was a beating I will not soon forget. Your professors knew that both life and care planning happen quickly on the floor.

Instead of all those hours in front of the chart, your awesomeness will be in front of the patient; where you should be in the first place.

So just give it a quick thought as you are gathering information and flipping through the chart. Soon enough into your first job you will be care planning before the shift report is even done. Trust me on this, it happens.

Keep this template in your mind (or paper if needed) to guide your choices.

What actions will you take today that will say, 'hey, mister patient man, I recognize you are having some issues with_____ and since you are important to me, I plan on keeping you safe by_____and I am planning to

*help you recover from your illness using these
actions_____.'*

Using goals as a focus point for your patient care is awesome. It is just likely that the goal will be much broader than it was in school and it certainly will not have a measurable time paired with it beyond getting to the goal in the 12 hour shift. Let those goals help your patient feel a sense of control in this strange environment. Always involve them if possible because what you think is important that shift may not be what the patient feels is important.

As long it is not an essential function there is always room to compromise, right? Work your plan to find the middle ground that will make you both happy.(**Note to Self**: patients get happier when they get control.)

You will most likely have no issues letting go of the need to produce a detailed map of goals, problems and interventions the way you needed to in school.

Focus Point: You know how to care for your patient. You don't need to write it all out. Trust yourself to provide awesome care and enjoy the extra time with your family the night before your shift.

Action Step: Email an old instructor and express your thanks for drilling care plan data in your head

Mantra Mojo: *The past cannot be changed it can only be accepted and learned from. I easily learn from it.*

Dear Wonder-filled human disguising as a nurse-

I know it is a lot to
take in..

you are doing more
than great with it
all..trust me on this
one..

Keep your head
down +   going

Keep going...........Keep going

It will get easier

Love you-

The future me

MIND YOUR MANNERS

Follow me here for a minute, okay?

One of my very favorite foods is green beans. I began my love affair with green beans at a young age. Very Marion Cunningham style, we had them every Monday + Thursday when I was growing up. My mom used Del Monte. Sometimes we got French style while others, they were swimming in cream of mushroom soup + little crispy onion thingy's on top.

No matter the exact presentation they were always from the can.

What in the Sam Hill does a can of green beans have to do with your transition to your floor or unit?

Well, actually plenty.

I grew up with those green beans in a can. That was just the 'right' way to enjoy green beans. It never occurred to me there was any other way because my mom's green beans were perfect.

You 'grow-up' in the nursing world with the thoughts, ideas and opinions of your professors and your school. Right or wrong, you measure everything that happens in the actual nursing world against what happened to you in school. Even if you had a crazy teacher with antiquated ideas on nursing, that is what sticks in your head.

You have no other frame of reference.

Like me and my green beans. My moms, in the can, were my only experience.

School sets the tone for your whole nursing career and you come to view the foundational information provided in school as the standard against which all other information is measured. You will come to look at the rules and traditions your professors teach as 'the only way' to do certain things in order to be a 'great' nurse.

Of course, that is not the truth. You will not see that as you step out into school though. You will be attached to these ideas from school, like I was my green beans, because it is 'just the way things are done'.

I don't recall the exact moment when I met the vine-fresh version of my little buddy the green bean. My vegan buddies described them as 'Mecca' for the green bean lover. My first thought?

These are disgusting! They do not EVEN taste like MY green beans. It was not love at first bite.

I can recall the exact moment I first judged another nurse, that moment of disgust for actions that were utterly and shockingly unlike the foundations I had learned in nursing school.

I was visiting a different floor as part of my preceptor training. She was giving medication to a sickle cell patient that was a frequent flyer and crazily annoying.

She walked in the room, did not speak, gave the narcotic without a single swipe of alcohol over the IV port, without a check of respiratory status, without diluting it at all or flushing the 3 inches of j-tube extension attached to it and left the room without closing the clamp on the line.

I was so attached to my way of doing things that I stood there, mouth open, in shock at the errors I just witnessed.

Much like my first taste of fresh beans, I was disgusted.

You will do this a lot these first few months of your nursing career because you are used to the way your school did things, aka the way your green beans taste. Right or wrong, they are the only things you know as you start your big gig at Smiley General. Seriously, the first time you see someone spike an IV bag of normal saline and throw open the roller clamp until all the bubbles escape along with 30 cc's of saline instead of carefully 'thumping' the bubbles while holding the tubing upside down without wasting even 1 cc, you will gasp.

If your school taught you to dilute IV push medications, the first time you see a nurse give an undiluted dose of medication to a patient, you will be downright offended!

The first time you count only to 2 while watching another nurse scrubbing the medication port on an IV access point, you will damn near short circuit.

The first time you watch a nurse give an IVP medication through an existing IV tubing port before checking the compatibility with the drug running in it already, you will be thinking...

'Someone is failing their skills test!'

The first time you see an experienced nurse push fentanyl, versed or some other narcotic in about a second, you will think, 'Slow down there missy you are gonna kill the patient!'

I am not even joking here. You will see it and you will be freaked the hell out by it. Try to breathe. Here is the thing;

Your instructors need you to be a SAFE nurse, right?

NCLEX tested your ability to keep people alive, right?

It is all well and good that you have a mini-panic attack when you see something that is not so safe happening.

You should continue all the things that school taught you. They are evidence-based and safe.
As I moved through the first year it kind of felt to me like the newbie nurses help the seasoned vets review their habits and the seasoned vets helped the newbie's with things to make them faster and well, just about everything else.

If you are prone to drama then figure out how to cover up the look of disgust on your face and figure it out quickly. Lose the need to correct your new peer group in front of anyone else, please.

Chat in private about it if you must and don't assume you saw something wrong just because you're not familiar with a technique.

Drop the thought that makes you 'right' and the other nurse 'wrong'. Remember there are many varieties of green beans.

To put it very bluntly here, mind your manners.

Do not come into their house telling them how 'wrong' they are.

Example: I once saw a nurse with 30 plus years experience stick a needled-up 10cc syringe into the end of a bag of saline to pull out the flush for the narcotic they were about to give instead of walk back to get one from the Pyxis..

I was sort of taken aback by it however; it worked and saved their feet the 50 yards; a fact which you will appreciate at the end of 12 hours.

Don't panic is the point here. There a lot of ways to perform skills and apply theory and the way you were taught is only one variation; not necessarily the one they learned; certainly not the only way to do thing. You get the point, yes?

Since higher education utilizes evidence-based teaching you can presume that your way is the most current perspective from an actual textbook. That is it.
Being all freshly-schooled makes it easy to get up on your high-horse and want to correct your co-worker that has been a nurse 15 + years.

Never.Do.This. Please.

As you read that sentence I know you thought, 'I would never do that, it would be like nursing suicide.' You will be tempted, I swear, because you want to fit in with this new group of people. You want them to accept you and one of the ways that can happen is for you to prove to them that you are a good nurse who actually learned something in nursing school. Showing off what you know will only annoy them and alienate you. You will need their help one day so keep your mouth shut here.

Nursing in the real-world does not happen in the vacuum of a school environment, you do not have 10 minutes to spike a bag of medication. So what are you going to do when you see things that are obviously not your can of green beans?

Just let other people have their own style of beans.

The best course of action here is to let go of any single

thought that you have about any other nurse and the way that they practice nursing. Do not judge anyone.

It is their practice, not your practice and besides, your own actions are the only ones that you can really control anyway, right? Makes a lot more sense to focus on you and you alone, right? Personally, I found this to be the kindest approach for all involved.

If you come onto a floor as the newbie and immediately start to tell the other nurses their technique sucks you are not going to make any friends. Old nurses do not take kindly to being told they are risking patient safety over a difference in interpretation of evidence-based practice. Trust me when I say that you are going to need friends much more than you need to hold onto your can of green beans.

That is not to say that you should ignore out-and-out dangerous activity. That goes without saying. You should always chat with the person that you saw engaged in that activity before you run to report them. Do it in private and keep it between the two of you. It may not be what you think you saw, after all.

If you can't stomach a chat with them about it try to find some creative way to remind them to use best practice.

That gal I saw give an IV push med without 'scrubbing the hub' first? Well, I didn't even mention it to her. The next time she went into the room I just handed her an alcohol prep pad right before the injection without a word. Later, she thanked me for helping her practice more safely, and for not rating her out to the boss before reminding her about it.

Once I got past my first months and had established myself

as a friendly, team-player that was interested in improving my own practice I started to ask questions about those skills I saw presented in a different way than I was taught. Some of the stuff on my list of things to ask were indeed just crummy habits of nurses that were overworked while some of them were actually short-cuts that did not compromise safety at all but gained me some extra time in the course of the shift. Lord knows I needed that time!

Be still for a bit and stay rooted in what you were taught. Your green beans are perfect for the transition into your practice.

Focus Point: Practicing the way you were taught, not any of the short-cut methods you see experienced nurses using will amp up your confidence and allow you to have those tough discussions with other nurses. You will learn so much from the experienced nurses around you, if not about medication administration and skills then certainly they will be excellent role models for how to manage your time.
Action Step: Write down what you see that you question. Ask questions at a good time to do that in private.

Mantra Mojo: *The only expectation of perfection is the one I place on myself. I will allow myself and those around me to be human today and every day.*

Dear Smarty Pants‑

Look, I know it is hard to watch things done so differently than in school. I know your brain is caught between wondering if
you should say something and wondering if you just spent 2 intense years learning the wrong way to do things.

Frustration is high..you know what though
Pat yourself on the back for just chillin out about it.

Good choice, you Closing your mouth and opening your ears is way more helpful in this time with your preceptor.

These people have so much knowledge, you need to soak it all up and be grateful they are offering to teach you.
Never mind the few peeps that you 'think' do things crazily+ dangerously wrong. Focus on your own practice. A phenomenal practice it is, might I add. Keep kickin butt! Me

142

TIME MANAGEMENT + MULTI-TASKING

Ah, the myth of the multi-tasking nurse.

It followed you from nursing school and has left you with some high expectations of your performance in these first months, no doubt.

Let's break this down for a second.

See, multi-tasking is a slightly deceptive term.

Plan ahead, yes. Anticipate needs, sure. Organize care in order to do one thing while on the way to another thing, totally!

Doing more than one thing at a time in the strictest sense is not something that any of us can do, truly. For some reason though, we throw this word around all over the place.

Sadly, I think most of us start our first nursing job with the thought that we outta be able to be an amazing + zenned out multi-tasker from day one. After all, we've spent the last few years engrossed in tons of things that all demanded our time and attention. We have succeeded at the learning, practicing, and testing on it, right?

Amazing, organized and zenned out are all great things to shoot for obviously and life in the fast lane as an actual RN is truly filled with competing priorities that you need to manage, juggle, and complete.

I'd like to ask you though to try to remove any preconceived notion of what multitasking will look like in the first months of your career. It is a sort of 'ramp up' thing. You get better as you gain experience and really only as you gain experience.

No matter how well you did this in school you will suck at it on the floor for a little while so remove the expectation of perfection here as you move into your new job. Take a breath and remember, you will get the hang of things it will just take more than a day to do it. *(Note to Self*: Feel frustrated and then move on-this is not a permanent condition.)

So somewhere in the first month of your 'actual' nursing career you are going to hear the voice of at least one of your instructors ringing in your head noticing each mistake you make and every little misuse of your time.

That voice you hear, well, it will be going on and on about all the things you are missing, at how unorganized you are, at how you 'should-be' *better* at this by now.

Stop, hold the phone a second.

Better in your first month? Really?

Tell that well-meaning voice to back-off.

Everything in school was connected to that pass/fail metric so this will be a place where you will start to freak out a little at your perceived imperfection. Like, you will be giving yourself an F in your head over how hard it is for you and how you have so many questions still.

But honestly, expecting yourself to be able to breeze into your shift 15 minutes early and feel prepared, to be caught up on charting throughout your shift, to give every medication and do every blood glucose check exactly on time, to be Johnnie-on-the spot when the doc calls and produce exactly the lab result or bit of info he wants at the moment, to be the perfect patient advocate and then to leave shift 15 minutes after it ends?

Nice goal but not so much reality for the first month, or six.

I have seen nurses that have been at it way longer than six months unable to leave shift on time. There is no way to know when some crazy thing is going to jump off and delay you. Things happen.

You know what I know for sure though?
That goal of doing everything on time (aka perfection), is in no way a realistic expectation to have of yourself from day one of your nursing career. You can keep it if you want to, it will just make for many a miserable drive home after shift. Using that time to remember the good you did will leave you much happier than beating yourself up for not being perfect, I swear.

That said, let's just take a minute and erase all of your preconceived notions about time management, multi-tasking and being an awesome nurse, please?

Press delete on the previous instructors recording stuck on repeat in your brain.

This may seem minor but its super-important work.

You will need a nice blank slate to start from if you want to retain the things you are learning + keep from losing your mind. Your professors meant well when as they instilled in you that being a good time manager was one of the essential characteristics of a great nurse.

All in all, that is a true statement however; school is where you get your feet wet. It is where you begin to learn about prioritization and delegation and how to put together the pieces of the big picture that becomes your shift. It is where you begin your apprenticeship as nursing time manager extraordinaire. Not where you perfect it.

No matter how prepared you feel as a student nurse, all bets are off the second you become an RN. Things change.

This is your show now, not your instructors or your buddies, it belongs to you. (*Note to Self*: Holy Crap, I am in charge of me!)
It is your career to craft. In a sense, even though you have been through clinical in school, you start from square one and it takes time to adjust. You have to be willing to give yourself some time.

For the love of Mike..give yourself some time!!!!

Unfortunately, there will be experienced nurses around you in this first month that have perfected this piece of our profession. This is bad only because it is human nature to use other humans and their behaviors to measure our own worthiness against.

The minute you catch yourself(and you will)admiring another nurse for how eloquently she whooshes around the unit doing so much at one time; just stop.

The second you hear that little voice in your brain that says 'you are never going to get this, you are a giant failure' (and it will); politely tell that voice to shut the hell up.

Seriously, measuring your worth as a new nurse by a standard that someone else is setting is detrimental to your psyche, remember? Comparing yourself to a fellow nurse with 5 plus years experience is enough to make you cry. Again, something I ask you not to do.

Comparison anywhere in your life will always suck the life out of you. You are unique and your learning process in this whole transition will be unique as well.

Stop wasting your time worrying you will 'never' get it. Trust me, you will, and much sooner than you expect.

I know so much about this myth because I was one of those people. Listening to the well-meaning professors and peers, I expected I would I juggle a lot of tasks at the same time, perfectly right out of the gate. I had done this in my previous corporate gig. I was a single mom for goodness sakes. I KNEW how to multi-task.

Add to this equation that I have a 'touch' of OCD when it comes to my work environment and 20 plus years of waiting to be a nurse under my belt, well, you can imagine that my expectations of myself were lofty, right? My first med pass as a nurse went something like this:

> Oh great! It is time to give morning medication. Super, I can do this no worries. A handful of oral meds, 2 IV piggybacks and a couple of IV push meds. My preceptor offers to help; I say "nope, I got this on lock."
>
> Time to show off that education, right?
>
> While I did look up all the medications for the labs needed
> + incompatibility as well as have a teaching in my head for the patient(who by the way was unconscious)I also forgot to crush the oral meds going in the NG tube before I got to the room, forgot to scan them before opening, forgot a bottle of sterile water, forgot the IV tubing for the piggyback, forgot to get a date sticker for the IV tubing after, forgot to bring the needle into the room to draw the med out of the vial, forgot the syringe, forgot the normal saline flush, forgot the alcohol wipes. Wow...

Yea, I am not lying one little bit. I made 9 trips out of the room before I even gave a single medication to my first patient that day.

How's that for time management? HA!

I made assumptions; that there would be needles, swabs, tubing and such in the room and I never checked for them at shift report. There had always been another nurse helping me gather things before, someone watching over me, guiding me and correcting me. Now with just the preceptor sitting back in the corner of the room it was a different thing. It was 'my' show...gulp!

The constant beep of the monitor asking me to take action was a 'little' distracting so I cut myself a tiny bit of slack. Even still though, I failed miserably at looking ahead that day. I did not anticipate what I might need through the process of giving medication. The rest of the day was pretty well a repeat of the above. By days end I had a list as long as my arm of reasons why I should have never become a nurse.

High GPA, ICU job right out of school and all...I sucked.

I spent most of the shift feeling embarrassed at my lack of organizational ability and pretty sure that my preceptor was chuckling silently to herself all day over it. Probably even telling the manager what a huge mistake they had made hiring me.

I got over it quickly though. Before I even made the drive home that night I realized that I needed to get off my own back and to let go of the thought that I could be perfect as a newbie; probably even ever.

There was this other thing I never considered that you might bump up against, too. In an effort to instill in me how important my job was, how many lives would depend on me, my school had made me terrified of making a mistake.

As in paralyzed, afraid to take any action because it might be the wrong one.

For example, I looked at the IV compatibility between 3 meds at least 5 times before I started the medication running. I was scared as hell that I was reading incorrectly. Really. After going back to the computer so many times my preceptor finally inquired as to what I was doing. She laughed hardily at my reasoning. She was like, ' Melissa, lexicomp is not going to update in the 60 seconds it takes you to start this med running, you know?'

Yes, I did know but I was hella scared.

I thought somehow that I was expected to be superhuman and never, ever, ever have a misstep in my actions. By the time I got home I could see the vise-like pressure that was putting on me.

I could see that over thinking every detail and setting the bar so high for myself was causing me emotional pain.

I could further see that I was setting myself up to fail with even a hint of the 'P' word in my noggin. That night, I resolved to do my best and trust that I would eventually develop into an awesome nurse.

A little harder for me was accepting that I was *not* going to be that awesome nurse on day one. I want to be a great nurse and in my head 'great nurses' have great time management and multitasking skills. My internal bar is super-high if you haven't learned that about me yet.

You may not admit this but I know you also hold some seriously high expectations for yourself. We are all here to save lives not harm them and we all take this responsibility seriously.

I spent some time that night laughing at myself and commiserating with a school friend. Thank goodness she was there to correct my belief that I should be performing like a seasoned vet rather than a new nurse.

The adjustment in thought my school buddy helped me with changed my thoughts a bit and I carried a new attitude into work with me the next day.

I even told my preceptor how I felt and she shared some of her most embarrassing first month stories with me. Imagine that? The phenom who was helping me had hesitated + made mistakes too. She even gave me some pointers on being prepared in advance. My ability to lay my ego aside, open up and to ditch my notion that I should be perfect, even for a tiny second, allowed me to accelerate my growth in this whole time management area. Most of that growth was related to my own expectations and assumptions. Once I fixed those a lot of things changed for me.
I used what I learned the first day and left that second day feeling much more empowered than I expected given how crappy I felt the day before. I was still knee-deep in suck but I could at least concede that I was not a horrible nurse

I have watched it go the other way too. Some of my peer group who are also new grads are still invested in the perfection expectation.

Know that you do not have to put this much pressure on yourself.

It is a choice.

I still get to work early but that is because I have a thing about being prepared and one of my biggest pet peeves is being late. These are personal preference not mandatory. I leave work on time. I stay so caught up most shifts that I ask my peers how I can help them before I ever sit down to chart and still leave on time. You can and will be here. You have to change a few things first.

1st and most important. Cut yourself a bit of slack. Allow yourself a damn learning curve, okay?

There is no prize for how much sleep you lose being worried about your job or for how many grey hairs you can gather as a new nurse.

Enough of me talking; here are some tried and true tips to help get you in your groove a bit faster. :
- Stop expecting perfection. It is not helpful thinking. At all.

- 86 your professor's definition of the 'perfect multi-tasking nurse'. Instead insert your own vision of where you should actually be at this point in your career.
- Find your own definition of multi-task. My vision is of a nurse with some foresight into what is coming, not a nurse who actually does more than one thing at a time. It is always best to define your shift on your terms and with your standards; no one else's.

- Learn to scan the room and the chart and think about the things you will need at the start of your shift. I used to pretend I got only one trip to the supply Pyxis per patient per day. Yea, a weird game to play but it really forced me to look ahead at all the medications and supply needs that this patient would have that shift. I left the room from my initial assessment with a written list of everything I would need from oral swabs to dressing change supplies, to chucks and everything in-between. Try it. You look a little like a pack-rat with your arms full going into the room but you save time like crazy; not to mention your feet. Plus, if those supplies are already in the room checking first keeps you from duplicating supplies which greens up the planet and eventually your wallet.

- Don't compare yourself to anyone anymore. Look at your co-workers as huge stores of nursing wisdom instead of measuring sticks of greatness to judge yourself against. In fact, use every chance you get to listen to the ones that are successful at organization and prioritization. Emulate them. There is a reason they are successful and still nurses after 15 plus years. Shhhh, don't tell my co-workers I am studying them, please.

- Leave your home life at home. Focus on your job while you are at your job. Your shift will morph into something amazing when you allow yourself to be fully present. In case you need further motivation to put down the facebook you should remember that you are opening yourself up to a ton of litigation if someone in your care should die and they can prove you were engaged with FB instead of the patient.

- Get to work early and get your patient assignment. Once you do take a minute and peek at their chart. Chart real-time. This will save you tons of time. It is hard to force yourself to do it when you are just learning. You will have to chart so you may as well do that while you are witnessing it rather than after you have been hard at it for 12 hours and want to go home. Trust me.

- Don't be afraid to ask for help if you need it or to say no when someone asks your help and you are overloaded. If you have extra time then by all means, love your neighbor and help. It's just that if you don't cultivate the habit of making your patients and charting the priority you will always be behind.

- Get in some habits. I am a Pisces and more of a 'go with the flow' than a 'habit' gal honestly but, in the nursing world I am all about the habitual stuff. That is because doing the same thing, in the same order every shift has saved my butt on the days that I am slammed because I don't have to stop and think if something was done. If it is part of the habit then I know it got done. Especially critical on those life-saving things like the stool for CPR.

- Volunteer to help everyone then observe carefully. I swear I have learned more time-saving tips from volunteering to assist those wise wonder nurses. Believe it or not there are ways to make a bed faster than you learned in school. Take some time and find the nurse that you see who spends most of their time out of the weeds. You know the one who is calm under pressure and almost always gets things done on time. Once you found them become a serious student of their mojo. Life. Saver.

I was lucky in that my last preceptor was one of those nurses. My other preceptors were good, this one though, he was phenomenal. I learned so much watching him work his magic. After almost a year of practice I could still fall into a great big bucket of shame and suck if I compared myself to him, instead I watch and learn. It never fails that every single shift I get to work next to him is better than 20 clinical days at school. There are a lot of nurses out there like him. Take some time and find one each and every shift. Study everything they do and keep what fits with your style of nursing.

Keep in mind that we are not shooting for perfection here, Nurse Awesome. *(Note to Self*: it is your practice not your perfect for a reason!)

If you actually use the above techniques instead of just read them in this book you'll start to feel less stressed quickly. You will still scrape your knees some but you will recover faster than without using them.

If you find yourself feeling particularly overwhelmed just stop and look honestly at where you are wasting energy with extra steps or where you are judging yourself too harshly.

Go back to the things up top and remember that you did not birth from the world of school as a nurse with perfected prioritization, delegation and time management skills. It will take at least 3 months to get your feet solid underneath you.

18 months in and there are still days when I am so busy that no amount of organizational skill will prevent me leaving the shift feeling wrung out and half close to crazy. That is the nature of nursing. Not all days are this way.

Focus Point: Experience is the best teacher. If you can approach each day with an open mind and maintain the ability to laugh at yourself and learn from your obvious lack of perfection well, you will learn more about time management in the first month than you did your entire nursing school career. I promise you can master it. I promise that will be soon.

Action Step: Watch your preceptor and incorporate one timesaving thing they do into your routine this week

Mantra Mojo: *I have plenty of time to do all I need to do*

Dear Amazing Nursing Awesome–

Whew, I know the last 2 weeks have been crazy and nothing like you expected. I am not sure why you're thinking you need to be able keep up with your preceptor on the first day. She has like a bajillion years of experience compared to

you so you are not going to be able to hang with her! Seriously, you have to cut yourself some slack. You are not supposed to know everything yet–no

one but you is expecting that, toots!

You are exactly in the place you need to be···take a damn breath already and relax..this is not school!!! I know you can't really feel it yet but I am telling you right now ···your medicine is magic

Big Love–Me

PS

YOU

ARE

AWESOME!

DON'T FORGET TO PEE

It is not outrageous to think that the people who become nurses also tend to be the nurturers of the world.

We are the folks in the crowd that stop + help when someone calls out. We don't just notice suffering; we take steps to stop it.

We are compassionate + empathetic. We are the band-aid of the world and typically we are pretty proud of it.

Unfortunately, we are not always as great at showing ourselves the same levels of compassion + tender loving care.

Some folks think that all nurses are a 'little' co-dependent. Others assert that we are secretly narcissist's who only take care of patients as a way of boosting our own importance in the world.

Whatever...

My theory is that we love the world so much that we often lose sight of how much energy we give away in the process of loving it until we find ourselves in the place that there is no energy left for our own care and feeding.

By that time, we don't really give a rat's tail about caring for our own needs we just want some sleep, a soft pillow and maybe a cookie.

Regardless, being able to put the needs of others above our own is pretty much the first line of the job requirement. Most nurses don't even sit down for a break until close to 6 hours into their 12 hour shift. Unless you count charting or peeing which technically do not count as a break! (**Note to Self**: no one will force you to take your breaks, you gotta claim them!)

How many professions brag about the amount of self-torture they can endure? As a newbie I was always hearing someone or the other brag about the time since their last meal or their last bathroom break as if it were some sort of prize they have won.

I always stop them with this really crazy look on my face and tell them I am certain their kidneys do not appreciate being ignored while muttering what a bad example they are setting for us newbie nurses under my breath.

Ours is a unique position that needs an equally unique solution because the vulnerable populations we serve need help when they need help; regardless of how full our bladder might be.

I know, I know, it is not like you can say 'you are going to have to wait one more minute for your medication mister seizing-man because I need to pee.'

This is not what I mean. You need to anticipate your needs and plan time for them just like you plan time to give patient medications. Seriously, plan breaks while you are planning care.

This is an area that you absolutely must address as you make your way into the real world. It needs to be part of your foundation. You need solid plans to provide yourself with excellent self-care while you learn to negotiate the space between shifts, the stress of 12 hours on your feet, and the myriad of other mazes you will be winding through as a beginner nurse. Exhaustion does not help your brain function. Sometimes making simple choices are difficult when you are depleted. Try to keep yourself out of that place.

Don't underestimate the power in a simple home cooked meal or an extra hour of nap to keep you from burnout or overload.

I work night shift and I used to try to take a nap the morning after my 3 night work jag. Not anymore. I just stay up until the evening and go to bed early the night after my shifts because I know that naps throw me into a total tailspin sleep-wise that take me days to recover from wholly. I have friends that need a 2 hour catnap that morning and are good to go. Pay attention to how you feel these first few months. Consciously listen to the signals your body sends when it is tired and then when it is bone tired. For me, when I start to get the chills out of nowhere in a warm room it means I am bone tired. I put it in park as soon as possible after this happens. If I do not then sickness is the next thing and I do not have time to be sick!

Increased or decreased energy and changes in your overall attitude are big signs trying to point the way to the better self care. Pay attention now are your body will force you to pay attention later.

It is all well and good for you to place priority on your patients' health however; your health needs to be equally important! Start here and build your own list of self-care essentials.

I have come to view these as my non-negotiable life items.

Sleep: Know your own sleep requirements-How many hours can you get by on in a pinch? How many hours do you need to function at your highest level? No matter what is going on for you, find a way to meet your minimums. Don't underestimate the way sleep resets your brain and heals your soul.

Rest: Know the signals your body sends when it needs break- Does your face breakout, do you develop a ravenous and ridiculous appetite for sugar? Are you the captain of crankiness when you are getting overwhelmed? Pay as close attention to yourself as you do your patients here. If something different is going on don't dismiss it. We all have a unique sign that we know to interpret as our body screaming for us to stop and rest. Listen to it. If you are unsure of how to determine your own sleep needs ask someone close to you to help you. All they really have to do is pay attention to your tone of voice, how much laughter they hear from you, how they observe you eating and how much you want to be engaged in life. Tell them you need them to help be your gauge until you get the hang of interpreting for your own self. Most of the important folks in our lives are happy to help!

Fuel: Feed yourself well. Take your lunch with you to work. Eat some damn vegetables and fruit. Carry a jug of water and drink it before you reach for coffee. Leave the chocolate on the break room table alone. It is tempting to 'fit in' and eat out with everyone when they order out. The sugar rush and the carb fix are short-lived but the change in your waistline is not and the truth is that crappy fuel in will give you crappy performance.

Activity: Exercise. Yea, no duh, right? We all know that regular sun and exercise is what helps our body thrive. It aids in metabolic process and releases feel-good hormones in the perfect amount. If you are counting the thousands of steps running up and down your unit as exercise please think again. You need focused time to get the benefits. Even if all you get is a dance break on the way from the shower to the car, turn up the tunes and dance, baby!

Attitude: I am repeating myself with this whole perfection thing I know, it is important, you must let go of the need for perfection. We don't think about this as being one of the stressors but man, considering the push to be perfect that school hurls at us daily it is easy to keep on expecting perfection from yourself. Asking yourself to perform without flaw or misstep puts a burden on your shoulders that no human can carry for long. There are fail-safes in place, allowing yourself to learn is not the same thing as allowing careless behavior it merely asserts what we all know already; none of us can be perfect. Let go of the need to be right. This is just another ego-based way of thinking that we bring from school. It can become a large chip that causes you to walk around ready to fight anyone and everyone that threatens to know it off if you don't let it go. You will learn a lot more and have a lot more fun without this need anyway.

Partners In Crime: Find some friends to share the journey with please. There are some things that only nurses understand. Bless your partner's head, they will grow tired of trying to figure out why you both love and hate your job.

Stress: Do something to release your stress every single day. Exercise, paint, meditate; whatever. You have to make a practice of letting it go intentionally or the days will dog-pile on you quick. No sense becoming a patient so fast. Find something you love to do and do it.

Disengage on the daily-so important that it got its own chapter later.

Note to Self: Uber-important to let it go!

It is easy to let the 12 hours run you instead of the other way around. It is not easy to find a way to assert some control in a world where your customers' life depends on speedy service. It is not easy to learn to process stress in a way that is productive.

I am going to say something now that is going to be hard to accept. Within the nurse-patient relationship, the most important person for you to take excellent care of is you.

It is a bold claim. I know it to be true like nothing I have ever known to be true before.

There is not any way that you can sustain a career in nursing for long if you are ignoring your own needs in favor of your patient.

There is not any way that you will stay healthy if you do not provide yourself with excellent care.
There is no way that you will enjoy your work if you are only giving to your patient and not giving anything to yourself.

I want you to incorporate these thoughts into your world. They are important. They are not easy but they are essential. You don't have to stop taking care of yourself to be a great nurse!

Focus Point: Figuring out how to take great care of yourself is just as s important as learning CPR only the life you save will be your own.

Action Step: Plan your breaks this week while planning patient care and stick to those times. Put yourself first at least once a shift. Begin to see self care as a non negotiable area of your life. Once you figure out what you need to do not give it up!

Mantra Mojo*: I am deserving of nourishment and rest.*

GPA ASIDE

Walking into your first shift as a nurse is exciting, no? You have spent so much time and energy working towards this goal and here it is finally. You are a nurse! Not only do you have a brand new uniform but you've got a brand new job, a sparkly new attitude, a brand new license and you are ready to heal the world!

Awesome!

There will be some other feelings accompanying you on the walk into your new nursing gig on that first day.

The elation of 'Holy cow, I'm finally a nurse', may be buddied-up next to a voice that says, 'What the heck am I supposed to do now?'

It is a bit like putting together a 1000 piece puzzle without the picture from the box. You technically have all the pieces but where exactly do you start this whole 'being a nurse' thing anyway?

I mean, I knew how to be a really kick ass student nurse. I knew I was becoming a nurse and the 'becoming' was a comfortable role. The 'being' a registered nurse, well that was all new to me.

School makes us spend a ton of time in the becoming phase. We wrap energy into learning the art of the NCLEX question, the expectations of clinical professors, and the technicalities' within this career we have dreamt about for years.

There is usually a brief class towards the end of your time in school that you might think will teach you about the first

163

steps to take once your feet finally hit the floor of your new job. Not so much. That class is designed to get you looking at growing into a more highly trained and educated nurse. It exposes you to a little bit of management woes and hospital politics but it will not answer the question...

What do I do next?

Nursing school taught me to do what I needed to do to pass those classes and clinical and gave me some critical thinking skills that I used while in a controlled setting. Key word; controlled.

This is easier that it seems at first blush. Treat your shift like a giant NCLEX question. Prioritize. What is most important?

You'll bat this ball around in your head a few times then conclude, well. Go and be a nurse, of course.

I surmised that I could use the same skills I did in school once I was out here in the trenches. What school did not do was prepare me for the 'unleashed on the world' feeling I had on that first day of employment.

It is natural to feel overwhelmed. Remembering to breathe helps!

I did well coming out of huddle up and shift change report but then I got to my patient assessment and just sort of froze. I did that slow blink...blink-thing where I looked around at the room and wondered, 'what the hell do I do next?' Now, don't misunderstand. I had the steps of what to do next down cold. I had practiced them in my sleep a million times. But standing there, actually in it for the first time, well now that was a horse of a different color.

Maybe that lack of trust in my own judgment was collateral damage from using so many brain cells in school or studying for that NCLEX or perhaps it was just a little bit of overwhelm.

All I knew was that the ability to make a choice about your patient and jump confidently into action to make things happen is a required skill for the ICU. I needed to gain confidence and gain some fast. ***Note to self***: stop doubting yourself so much!

My first thought? Prop myself up with my grade point average or the officer duties I held in school. Maybe I could glean some edge from the professional experience I had as a department director in my past life or use some of the problem-solving skills I developed as a single mom. Truth was, I pulled from all those areas all the time anyway so there was no special edge there.

Harsh reality here, no one cares what school you went to or that you graduated in the top 5% of your class.

No one wants to hear what awards you won or what office you held in school.

If you try to tell people your GPA you are just asking for trouble; expect some laughs at your expense.

As someone that worked her ass off to maintain a high GPA while working + serving as an officer in school this was a hard pill to swallow. No doubt the work of my ego again. (***Note to self***: most things in life are better if you lay ego aside.)

All they want to know is that you can nurse.

They want to know that you understand disease process.

They want to know that they can count on you to have their back and most importantly they want to know that when shit hits the fan and a patient is crashing that you will not seize up. They want to know that you know what to do in crisis; not in class.

Most likely this is exactly what will happen the first time you face a true emergency or critical decision about your patient care. Expect a bit of deer in the headlights feeling. Know that it passes quickly.

You are treated differently as a peer than when you are wearing that 'student nurse' badge. I was lucky enough to be able to spend my last month in school on the same unit I work on now so these people knew I had just graduated.
In my mind that meant that I was still not qualified to participate in RN discussions fully and would be able to sit in the safety net of 'student' a bit longer. I thought I would be eased into practice and that no one would be asking me for advice or expecting me to make decisions about patient care or giving report to doctors from the jump. I expected there would be that 'student' cloud hanging over me for at least the first 6 months.

Turns out, those 2 little letters carry some special kind of mojo with them because to my new peer group I was 'one of them' from day one.

Day one I tell ya. Day. One.

Part of me appreciated this professional respect and another part of me was like, 'what the hell are you people thinking I am NEW at this'.

While I was new, I was a nurse not a student. I thought this was just my unit however; most of my nursing peeps experienced this same thing. They were treated as equals the first day they stepped foot on their new jobs. You should expect it, too.

This is a bit of an adjustment and a bit unnerving since you have spent so much time in the student role. It will help if you can bask in the sense of pride you felt for passing the NCLEX when you start feeling like you should not be their peer, because yes indeed you should.

It may take a minute to flip it in your head from student to registered nurse. The first months are the time to do it. The biggest adjustment for me was the fact that you don't have to clear your plan of care with anyone else or ask permission before you turn a patient or do oral care or any of those other nursing orders that are in your control. No one will be standing there to nod approval of your choices. It is all you.

You're in control, be prepared for this, it is going to be a bit of a shock but it will feel amazing too!

While your new peer group will look for you to be an RN not student it will take some time to prove you can do this job, both to yourself and the nurses on your floor. They will not so much police your activity or approve of it as act like a safety net when they see you have fallen.

I have no doubt that you can do it. It is not all that different than tackling care plans or giving that first injection so many moons ago and you sailed through that task.

Adopt an attitude of being a hard worker and it will happen much more quickly than if you come in with the attitude that because you were the smartest person in your class you will be the smartest person on your floor.

Probably the best choices I made as a new nurse was to be the person that never spoke about GPA and the person that never sat down until everyone on my side of the unit had been assisted if needed. Both have helped me gain friends and gain knowledge, fast!

So how can you gain some confidence as you grow into the nurse you see yourself becoming?

First off,

Don't panic yourself if you feel really lost on the floor. Pay attention to your self-talk. If you find yourself using words like <u>always</u> and <u>never</u> to describe your day then take this as a sign that you are catastrophizing in your mind. Take a step back and regroup. You are letting your imagination and fears get the best of you. Stop it, just stop it.

Second, start looking for someone on your floor that you can trust to give you feedback on your skills. Look to them to be your ground point or check point when you start to get wrapped up in the negatives mentioned in the first step above. Tell them, 'I really feel like I suck at (insert task here)and I would really love it if you could watch me do it and tell me what I can improve' They will help.

Third, stay in the present moment. Don't relive mistakes you made in clinical or skills lab. Fail that Foley test? Suck at IV starts? Forget it! You will go nuts by allowing some ghost from skills lab past to haunt you in your present patient situations. On my second day of work I was unable to insert a Foley on a patient. The self-flogging I gave myself in that moment of defeat was horrific. I was so embarrassed, that is, until I saw an experienced nurse also having trouble with that patient's anatomy.

Fourth, keep your eyes open for the things you are finding yourself feeling wonky while doing. The things that make you silently hope no one just saw how much you hesitated before you did them. Do them a lot. You will get better with repetition. When I started this was IV starts for me, I would hit about 1 out of 5 on the first stick. Most people think that an ICU nurse can hit a tiny vein on even the most dehydrated patient and so they call ICU to do the hard sticks. Funny thing is that most of our patients start off with peripherals but end up with central lines so we do not start as many IV's as the general world things. I had to ask for help at first. You might even pick a few of these things that you have 'almost' mastered, you know the things you did in school that you will likely need to do over and over again on the floor then set about the task of intentionally practicing so mastery comes more quickly.

What areas did your self-assessment in the 3rd chapter reveal to you that you need to practice? Your implementation plan for yourself should include these things so you can build confidence. Things to focus on:

Spiking and priming IV tubing
Interpreting lab values and knowing the reason they are important
What does high K+ do? What does high NA+ do?
How are you with checking residuals in an NG tube? Crushing medications and using the NG for administration?
Do you communicate in a productive way?
Can you organize your day?
How comfortable are you if you need to assist with procedures?
Can you gown and glove while maintaining sterile field?
What procedures are done on the daily in your unit?

If you work on a cardiac floor chances are you need to know a lot about CHF and teaching for this disease. Do you? If not, take the initiative and learn it.

Are you on a post-partum floor? You should know the how to 'feel' the difference between a firm fundus and a boggy one as well as a million other OB specific things that school just touched on. I am not talking about the book specifics here Nurse Awesome, but the actual applications of the specifics, learn them.

Are you in the ICU? Better beef up your skill with those ventricular drains, ventilators and chest tubes before you start.

When you take a skill you mastered and put it in an actual patient situation it can make you fumble and feel stupid. Don't let it. For example, an IV start on a dehydrated patient is much different than a pregnant woman. An NG tube insertion looks a lot different on a calm awake person than on an overdose patient that is literally fighting you each step of the way. Sterile dressing change is one thing in the serenity of school lab; how do you change that dressing and maintain sterile field when your patient cannot cooperate at all with the procedure?

I know these all sound like little things and they are really. But these are little things that add up to make a big difference for the way you feel as you walk out onto the floor every day.

If you project confident and calm energy in front of you then you will create a better working space than if you were in a general funk because of what you do not know.

Take control here. Remember, it is your career.

Once you establish some basic stuff in that first month, start to examine the loot in your bag of tricks for BIG situations, you know those where you cannot hesitate, new nurse or not.

Start here, Nurse Awesome!

You just have to know what to do because you have about 60 seconds before some real damage happens. Try these out:

> Patient c/o of new onset chest pain/ shortness of breath
> Seizures
> Fall precautions
> Stroke Screening/Dysphagia Screening
> Flash Pulmonary edema/Cardiac Tamponade
> Patient is non-responsive
> ECG changes
> When do you do CPR and when do you shock?

There were a lot in my specialty area of ICU. Are there some knowledge areas that you should beef up on in your specialty area? Take a minute and list them:

I will admit it does suck a bit to have worked so hard at that GPA to find that not one single person will ask you about it. I totally wanted someone on my new floor, at least one other nurse, to ask me what mine was so I could prove to them that I had the goods to be an equal player in their world. It wasn't so much the GPA that meant anything to me, it was the work that went behind it and the fact that I believed it sent the message that I 'belonged' on the floor with my amazing new peer group.

Get this though; they actually *can* see your GPA. You show them by knowing your patients + taking excellent care of them. You prove it by anticipating needs, preventing complications with your sharp nursing judgment and critical thinking skills. Once I realized this I lost the need to show anyone my GPA. Amazingly enough once I was able to let go of the need to 'prove myself' I began to gain a lot of confidence those first few months in this new, non-safety-netted place.

Taking some time, making a plan, letting go of your past mistakes, not to mention setting realistic goals is the way to start building confidence in this new world. Obviously, taking an active role in your own career and skill set can be quite empowering and worth every moment of effort spent building your arsenal of awesome.

I want you to feel proud of the work you have put into this career. It matters. You matter.

Focus Point: Bring the same love of nursing and people into your first job that you brought into school. Take responsibility for the energy you bring to the workplace and make choices that demonstrate appreciation for your new friends will open communication paths and keep you from feeling like you are being 'eaten'.

Action Item: Do not speak of your GPA.

Mantra Mojo: *What I put out is what I will get back. I choose to put out positive thoughts and good wishes*

DO NURSES REALLY EAT THEIR YOUNG?

I heard this phrase so much the last 2 semesters of nursing school, it wore me out. I could not imagine why anyone that chose to care for sick, injured and dying people would be cruel to me or anyone else for that matter.

The answer in my head to that question was 'of course they do not eat their young do not be ridiculous!' Unfortunately, the reality is that sometimes it feels like they do. I wouldn't spend a lot of energy worrying about it, despite what you have heard. This is an easily changeable area that has a ton to do with your own actions and attitudes.

My first reaction to learning this was one of disbelief followed quickly by a whole lot of laughter. I still use laughter to deal with it.

While I could see that this may indeed be an issue with some folks, it certainly seemed like an easy enough issue to solve.

Aggressive behavior happens everywhere, not just in nursing. It can be particularly intense in a setting where you battle the angel of death every day. The current nursing culture playfully, perhaps nervously, named this aggressive, take no bullshit approach as 'nurses eating their young'

I think it is a reaction to several separate things.

Nurses are busy y'all. They have zero time to spare in dealing with the shenanigans of a newbie. While you may be an awesome nurse the nurses around you do not know that yet. All they know is that any shenanigans you create they will have to help you fix. That takes some time they already are

173

running short on, you know?

Mix a bit of fear that you may hurt their patient, which affects their license and a bit of fear in that you know all the latest stuff and that you may replace them. No wonder they throw off a hostile vibe to us newbs so often, huh?

Until we change our culture totally and create a space where these experienced nurses have plenty of time to assimilate us into the goings-on of the floor and where they do not feel afraid, you are going to deal with some of this whole stupid thing.

Just stand up for yourself calmly + confidently. Act like a competent + capable nurse that you are and your new peer group will be more apt to help you and less apt to eat you.

The whole notion sounded ridiculous to me because no matter how I connected the dots there was not one single way I could picture me, as a new nurse, to be even a tiny threat to one who was experienced.

I mean, seriously people. Why would there be fear
when you looked at me or my peer group? We have
zero experience as nurses.

No way, no how that anyone might be threatened by me (
Note to Self: maybe they are only annoyed by the constant sunny attitude you carry. Turn it down just a notch.)

My first experience with this changed my viewpoint somewhat and brought me to a place of profound sadness mixed with a heaping dose of anger. I was a student and we were mid-way through the first semester of school in afternoon post-conference. I was happy the shift was over. One of my peers was not smiling instead; she was on the verge of tears as she shared the details of her shift from hell.

She had been paired with an outspoken and strong-willed nurse, quite the opposite of her own temperament. This nurse, she was not the least bit interested in being buddies with a nursing student. She did not love teaching but loved that extra preceptor pay. She was accustomed to running a tight, quick shift without time to backtrack, explain or help a needy nursing student with the myriad of things nursing students need help doing.

It sucked because my friend had looked forward to this shift. She invested time learning about her complex patients, reviewed the skills she would use and showed up with a willingness to work hard and be taught well. She looked for this more experienced gal to guide her and all she got was trashed. Although she held up her end of the deal there was no reward for her efforts. Instead, she spent the day being reminded that she was 'just a student'; being corrected abruptly and told her evidenced-based practice was not at all practical in the real world. She was also showered with more than her fair share of dirty glances and rolling eyes coupled with an occasional condescending remark in front a patient as an excuse for the delay in medication administration.

I listened but tried to keep an open mind because this was only her perspective. Maybe my peer had done a horrible job. Maybe she was overreacting.

As I sat searching my brain for possible good explanations of what I felt was an abusive situation my friend had endured, my instructor began to explain. This was 'normal' behavior and something we would need to get used to if we were to survive in this world. We needed to 'toughen-up' and learn not to be so sensitive. We needed to take the lesson and grow from it and understand that 'everybody does this' to some extent in this field. She did not seem all that surprised by the experienced nurse's actions. I knew my instructor better than this; she had a heart. I think offering defense of the staff nurse's horrible and unprofessional behavior just became a norm of sorts. Something done without thinking.

I left that day with a belly ache, appalled at how the word 'everybody' just rolled out of her mouth. No second thought, no inkling of needed change. Since when is it okay to treat someone like crap; regardless of the situation? Why was it okay to berate someone or question their intelligence and credibility with no proof? Would this be tolerated in other careers? Why was it okay in medicine? The week before in theory class we were told that nursing was one of America's Most Trusted Professions? Really?

I wondered whether America would still trust us if they knew that we treated one another badly while we took care of them? I was shocked that there is an expectation within nursing culture that older nurses 'eat' their young and that nothing is really done to address it. Learning that this was one of those 'rite of passage' type things you are just expected to endure, like frat-house hazing, and then pass on to new nurses yourself was total nonsense to me.

The activist in me wanted to fix it right then and there. I wanted to demand a better standard in school + in those clinical situations. I guess my advanced age made me know better. Nursing school offers it own share of battles that have nothing to do with this one. If I jumped off feet first into trying to make people act nicer I was in for a huge fight. My energy was better spent absorbing care plan data than trying to re-parent grown folks. So, I just hung on for the ride in school, focused on the point of my time there and knew that I would eventually get a chance to change things by example with my own behavior when I precepted a new nurse.

Turns out making a conscious choice to stay off the 'be nice' band wagon did not make me stop seeing it. I noticed it in other places too.

In school as professors pressured students to be 'perfect' in ways that verged on abusive, between cliques inside my nursing program and I continued to see it in clinical situations. While it left me angry I had honestly all but erased it from my memory bank once school was done until I saw it between two of my peers at that brandy-new hospital I call home.

These two nurses I work with, they are both phenomenal. Kind + strong in heart and skills, these two have nursing chops for days. They take quiet and confident control of any space they enter; no matter how chaotic that space might be at the moment.
In ICU it is pretty damn important to take control; and these gals do! I am in such awe of them that I leave every single shift I work with them feeling as if I should pay them something for the 12hour tutoring session I just received.

I noticed one day that I was being asked to come to the other end of the unit to cosign insulin by one of these phenoms when the other one was sitting two feet away. There was palpable friction. They were avoiding each other like crazy and it surprised me. They were so much alike in both heart + smarts I wondered if they could even see that in one another. No doubt there were unexpressed issues, maybe a bit of jockeying for position in the unit or maybe one of them felt threatened by the other.

I could have cared less about this 'experienced nurse' version of the whole eating your young thing. They were both incredible nurses and humans which made it hard for me to understand how each of them missed seeing the awesome reflection of them in the other, really. Thankfully they worked it out eventually. In the process though, they let me see that the passive-aggressive behavior crap isn't reserved for new nurses.

Their struggle gave me a better perspective. It didn't just happen to newbie's. Nurses 'eat' other nurses at all levels of the food chain.

Something that we need to look at more closely and change eventually. For now, just observe and don't get bogged down by it,

It comes more subtly from the higher up via their emails about this or that thing that absolutely must be done by such and such time *or else*, different package but same deliverable. Fear.

Force used to make you afraid in order to make you do something? It is total crap and something I hope will change through our collective efforts one day. Fear is not really the best way to motivate people. Give me something meaningful to learn, tell me why it is important and there will be no force needed.

That aside, I thought that all the motivation via fear was just going to be a nursing school thing. There is a lot in the way we treat each other in the 'real-world' that could use some TLC and all the possible variables can't fit into a neat little container. That is what makes this type of bullying so tricky.

It looks different based on your place in the circle. If you are management you can't see your pointed emails punctuated with exclamation marks as threatening, if you are those experienced nurses you cannot see your eye-roll or attitude as demeaning and if you are the new kid on the block you cannot see your detail-oriented, sunny + excited behavior as annoying.

A profession centered on caring should learn how to care for its own first, don't you think?

So, where the hell do we start?

Your choices, of course. Don't get lost in the muck of it all this first month. You have plenty of other foundational-type work to do.

Just make the conscious decision to be mindful of your thoughts, words and actions. That is a great place to start. Refuse to participate in the battles + do not gossip.(**Note to Self**: go over your safety checks in your down time instead of playing ego games.)

Need a few more floaties to keep you above water until your feet find the bottom in your new world?

>Treat people on your new floor the way want to be treated. Isn't that the simplest thing ever? You are responsible for the energy you bring to the space so, take responsibility for your actions. If you offend someone; apologize. If you come off bad then admit it and change it.

>Be mindful of your contribution +check yourself daily, If you are not contributing positive to the environment then change something.

>Don't walk onto the unit with your evidence-based practice blazing and ready to correct all the wrongs you see in other peoples practice. Keep your eyes on your own practice. Look, I get this. It isn't that you want to correct anyone; maybe you have been a little overzealous in your attempts to fit in and show your

GPA. Just curb your dog.

Don't waste time with defensiveness or by contributing to the bullying. Listen to criticism, flip it in your head to a positive and take it as contribution to your craft. If you have been told you have a know it all streak take a step back and examine that statement then correct the misunderstanding or yourself.

Pay attention to how you feel. If you start to feel like you are being attacked or as if you are getting the cold shoulder from someone then be proactive about it. Passive aggressive bullshit is not helpful. Be direct and ask if you have pissed them off. Clearing the air makes space for better relationships to develop. Know it is not all about you. In fact, very little of it is about you at all. You are just the domino that sets off the chain reaction started somewhere else. You are the proof that mgmt hates them, that they are old, that they can be replaced. As nonsensical as that sounds, it is painfully true.

Recognize experienced peers as a source of inspiration and show them respect-Society sucks in the way it pits people against each other to begin with-being a fairly competitive person myself I have had to work my way out of that place. Defer to their perspective if it seems right but always use your own brain too. Actively enlist their support. Notice what you admire about them. Do they do something with particular ease? Tell them, everyone likes to be reminded that they are awesome from time to time; including more experienced nurses.

Don't base your opinions on another person's experience.

Don't be nice to someone's face and then be shitty

behind their back—that is adding to the issue
Become a person that can be relied on by all the
nurses on your floor

Create healthy boundaries

Before you decide someone is being awnry try
putting yourself in the other persons place for just a
minute.

I always take the time to say something positive to
every person I speak with each night. Phrases that
start with, I appreciate you when. I respect that you, I
never thought of doing it like this, I admire your
experience...These go a long way to improve
relationships with even the most cranky people.

When you step out of your school uniform and into your work
scrubs for the first month you are surrounded by an air of
positivity that is palpable to the nurses who have been on the
job a while.

You are excited to be at work but that can be quite annoying
to the long-timer who is beat down by the system. The
patients and politics of the unit have not begun to suck the
life out of you.

Even though you have no thoughts that you could replace
anyone they might feel threatened because you are so shiny
and new. While you are in awe of what you see these
dynamos doing around you on the daily, they are in fear that
management will prefer your skill set over theirs; regardless
of their time on the job.

Some of this you cannot change. Let people be who they are,
some nurses just hate all the things that disrupt their day.
That is okay. Let them be pissy and give them a wide berth

around you, just don't contribute to their belief that you cannot be trusted with your crappy behavior or choices.

What can you control? Yourself, of course!

Pay attention to your own actions. Make sure that you are not being a know-it-all + make certain you mind your manners.

The minute you begin to wear that RN badge you become an integral part of the culture you inhabit. So, do not underestimate the power behind your own thoughts, words and actions.

The truth is there are benefits to being a brand new nurse. You do have certain swag about your step. You have spent the last few years learning all the latest and greatest evidence in patient care. That information and how it has shaped your practice is important. You are happy as all heck to be out of school while they may be struggling just to get to 'okay' each shift; let alone happy.

Don't be ashamed of your happy place, peanut. You earned it. Don't use it against the people around you like a weapon either. Do your job and let others do the same. They will learn from you and you will learn from them.

You are qualified and you have been called to be a part of this awesome profession. (**Note to Self**: qualified not prepared)

You will never have as much experience as the wise nurses we meet on our first job nor are you supposed to be that skilled just yet. I am not sure if there is a single answer for this issue. I see the only solution coming at it from all sides and starting at the point of entry.
That means you, Nurse Awesome.

I am not suggesting that you launch into a full scale mission to change the culture on your unit and ferret out all the bully-like behavior in this first 30 days. That would be dumb, huh?

I am encouraging you to take an active stand against it by making 100% sure your words and actions are not contributing to that negative standard. NO bullies or bullshit allowed in your practice!

I am not saying you can change everyone, obviously not.

I am saying that you can change yourself. We have to start there.

Focus Point: Be conscious of the energy you bring to every encounter. The transformation of our culture really does start with you.

Action Step: Find one thing good about every nurse you encounter this week and tell them how you how awesome they are-

Mantra Mojo: I will respect every nurse and their practices even if they are not like my own

TAKE 5...

5 questions you should be able to answer with ease

How can I make this better for myself or-take control of my own health? Am I going to die? Will this hurt? Am I getting better? What would you do if you or your loved one were in this situation?

5 absurd things you will hear from patients.

If you touch me I will file charges I am allergic to everything but dilaudid My doctor says I am the healthiest fat person he knows When can I go home, I have a doctor's appointment? I can't breathe (from the screaming patient)

PROTECTING YOUR LICENSE

This is a tough chapter to write. I don't like focusing on negative things, unfortunately negative stuff does exist. So while I would just as soon work from the place that says you don't need to be worried about losing your license as a new nurse; you absolutely need to be educated about the rule sets you must, must, must follow.

It would be hugely irresponsible on my part to not even bring it up.

There are a lot of situations that might cause you to come up before department management or peer counsel. I mean stuff you never even 'thought' would ever be questioned might very well be questioned. There are places you need to protect yourself that you might not realize.

If you have not read your states Nurse Practice Act, you should. If you have not looked at the Board of Nursing Rules and Regulations for your state, by all means you need to do that before you start to practice.

In Texas, where I live, the BON-RR is 188 pages. There is a lot of data to absorb and it is very specific. It intends to leave no room for misinterpretation of the rules. No one sets out to lose their license. The stories I have heard around my job suggest that people get here most of the time through either accident or addiction.

Think like a nurse was a phrase I know that you heard more than once. Thinking nurses always assess first, right?

They ask questions before, not after, they take action.

Nurses look forward to see the implication of their actions, they err on the side of caution and place patient safety up front and center always.

All the rules that are in place are there to ensure that you are thinking like a nurse before you take action, that your patient is safe, that you are going to keep people alive.

If you are having a tough time interpreting the rules then chat with some other nurses to see what they say about it. If you are still unclear then call the board. Seriously, it is that important for your future to be clear. They will chat with you at length about what they expect. Better to do that up front if you are hesitant than on the back-end when your integrity and license are in question, right? (*Note to Self*: ALWAYS ask questions if you are unclear.)

The other thing to consider here is what your facility rules are about the big things. What happens if you go on break and do not tell anyone? What if you leave without giving a shift report because the other nurse is running late? What time frame do you have between removing narcotics from the Pyxis and the time you give them? Can you draw multiple times from the same vial on the same patient? So if say you get a 2 mg vial of Ativan and use 1 mg the first hour can you use the other 1 mg in the next few hours or do you have to waste it and start over again? What is the policy on wasting controlled substances? What is the policy on overriding medications or getting them without the order attached to the patient yet?

What is the policy for nurses entering a physician's order? How do you document a phone order? Are there orders that are considered to be 'follow-through' or protocol orders? Learn how your facility wants you to do this and learn what the state you live in says about this piece. Lots of states in the

USA so there is no use going into it here.

Look up Safe Harbor; it is one of those things you need to understand before you go into a shift. If you have not peeked at your hospital rules regarding it or the BON rules in your state then please do so. It is too late to stop once you get into the shift. If you feel intimidated or coerced into taking an assignment you are not competent to take then you have fewer options. Be strong and say no if you need to do it. There is a unique challenge for new nurses. The nice nurses on your new unit will make the assumption that you know how to do 'most' nursing things. If you go to work on a specialty floor that is different, let's just say for the sake of discussion that this is a medical/surgical floor and the physician has asked you to assist with a thoracentesis, have you done this before? If not, please speak up. No one is going to be phased by it before the task. You can bet you will ruffle a few feathers if you wait until the doc is at bedside looking for a piece of equipment that you have not provided because you did not know any better. Speak up, the other nurses will help!

Another way to state this is just simply do not do things that you do not feel safe doing. There is no shame in claiming the fact that you are uncomfortable performing a skill. Better risk looking dumb because you do not know something than risk hurting a patient.

You heard this in school so many times so I know you know this; it is super-hard to 'risk' looking dumb so this is where your personal integrity comes into play. If you are scared to go to one nurse for fear of judgment then find someone else. Just do not risk your patient if there is ever an uncertainty that you can complete the task. Sorry, I am off my soapbox now. Here are the things you need to make sure you do so that none of the above happens:

- ✓ Do not sign for insulin that you did not see someone give-I don't care if it was 2 units Do not sign for a waste on a narcotic for someone if you do not see them waste it
- ✓ If you have the least bit of twinge in your tummy that something is not right then just do not do it. Trust your gut feelings!
- ✓ Just because a doctor asks you to do it, does not mean it is in your scope of practice. For example, intrathecal medication administration is NOT in your scope; even if Dr. Awesome says you are capable.
- ✓ Don't break the rules that you know are in place for patient safety-bed alarms and such..
- ✓ The floor as a whole is responsible for call lights not just one nurse so if one goes off and you can answer it than do it. You can be hauled into court if something goes wrong and you were on the floor when a call light went unanswered.
- ✓ Don't forget to report to the board if you change address + keep up with your CEU's
- ✓ Do not practice medicine. Always have an order before you do something to the patient or give something to the patient. Just because a doctor 'always' gives a fluid bolus to his patients when the blood pressure is low please do not assume he will this time around. Assumption is practicing medicine and you will lose your nursing license over it.

Just stand firm in what you know to be the evidence that serves to protect both yourself and your patient. Work with a large degree of integrity. If you mess up then say so, please. Following physicians' orders is a great place to start.

DOCTOR'S ORDERS

Did you leave school with the belief that you were fully equipped to read, interpret and follow up on any order that a physician might write for in the course of your shift? Man, I sure did!

This is 'mostly' a true statement. I say mostly because the application can get a bit tricky for us new folks. A more accurate assessment of interpreting physician's orders says that we are equipped to do it however; we need a ton of practice to feel like we are actually prepared for it. Like just about everything else we do this first month on our own.

You will not feel comfy and cozy with this area from day one on your floor. Don't sweat this much though because this is one of the easiest things you will have to adjust to and you do it a lot!

This is one of those places I felt the most discomfort with when I first went to work at Smiley General. I work in ICU and things are often done in a time-sensitive, hurry-cause-the-patient-is-about-to-die manner. That was a lot different than in simulation lab at school or in my time with preceptors in my clinical rotations. God forbid a theory test ever asks you to give a medication without an order first; not in a million years. It happens in ICU a lot. As in you anticipate your crashing patients needs, override the med in the Pyxis, then the doc holler out the order as he is prepping to do the emergent and life-saving thing, you are entering the order and another person is giving the med. This is a more accurate description. You need to know how to handle it in a way that protects yourself and your patient; because you are an awesome patient-protecting nurse.

My school did a great job teaching me to read a physicians order. I knew the differences between scheduled, standard protocol and as needed, or PRN, medications. I learned a ton of pharmacology so I knew the usual dosage and side effects of the drugs I would see a lot of in the field. Drug interactions and half-life's were no issue. I knew what things needed to be ordered by a doctor and what was considered a follow-through order that I could place based on a previous order. These were the logical and linear pieces and they are the easy parts. School helps you get super-good at following rules so once you learn the rules around physicians orders it gets easy, right?

While I was less than confident with my ability to interpret and follow all that the doctor may order. I certainly left school knowing the most important piece. I knew how to keep my patient safe while I protected my license. I knew what to do so that I would never, ever be accused of practicing medicine.

Nah, my challenge was here. See, the rules of logic and thoughts of protection often get tossed to the side when in the real world. A textbook definition of the flow of orders from doc to nurse was only that; textbook. I found myself saying to doctors, 'what? Wait, I thought that you would enter this order'.

I did this so many times in the first 30 days. I seriously got laughed at a lot until I realized I was trying to apply what I learned from the books to a variety of non-book situations.*(Note to Self*: be flexible, sunshine!)

The first time a doctor asked me to push the etomidate and fentanyl with a patient as he was standing at the head of the bed preparing to intubate the decompensating patient was NOT the best place to say, 'but there is not an order for those medications'. Luckily, another awesome nurse anticipated

190

the need and reached in her pocket for the medication before I had a chance to be ashamed.

I seriously thought that doctors entered all patient orders themselves because that was what the textbook taught? Silly huh, imagine my surprise after I waited an hour for an order to 'show up' in the MAR after I had spoken with the doctor about it. I called back to clarify that I was able to give the new medication, thinking I had misunderstood the order, since I didn't see said order entered by the doctor. Ass-chewed and lesson learned. He was waiting for me to enter it.

It smacked against everything that I had learned about the rules, you know? Nurses don't enter orders, right?

Worth noting here, there is a fair amount of critical thinking that goes into following a doc's order for a patient. This would be the place where you get to apply the skills you learned in nursing school; especially the ones you used on those test questions that left you with 2 answers that both 'seemed' correct. Only the question data that helped you pick the answer becomes the actual patient that you are carrying out the order on. This is when you will start to be grateful that your instructors pushed you so hard.

For example, your question in school may have been something about a patient going to get a CT with contrast that is also a diabetic and using metformin. The question gives you an elevated creatinine number and some kidney complications. You're asked to decide when it is safe for the patient to go to CT.

So now, put your thinking cap on; the question data in real-life becomes your patient assessment, their lab values, and the whole picture of that patient. Your prime directive is patient safety, right? So you pick how long to wait on that patient, talked to the doc about his need for the CT, ask if it can wait...you get the jist of this I am sure. If the creatinine is high and they are on metformin you could cause some serious kidney issues simply by failing to speak up and tell the doctor about it, yo!

So, first things first. Never just follow an order without thinking it through and looking at all the most current data on your patient, please.
Probably the simplest thing you can do to keep this from being an issue for you is to keep a focus on the 5 rights you learned in school and use this as a guide to practice. If something seems off to you in one of those 'rights' then ask questions.

Look at the parameters the doc gives you. If it is a drug that doesn't have a parameter but needs one you should call the doc and get some.

Do not though, look for literal enforcement of those rule 'nurses never enter orders' as you maneuver through the first month and don't be afraid to ask for clarification if you are wondering if the doc wants you to enter an order.

School provided a needed guide for patient safety. You will frustrate yourself beyond belief if you cling tight to those hard and fast rules when it comes to how doctor's orders are entered. Don't stand around stomping your feet waiting for it to be like school cause it just is not.

The second thing to keep in mind that will help to keep your frustration level down this first month, I guess that would be to know that verbal orders happen; a lot.

Yea, we are taught they should never happen but they do. Depending on the area of care you are in this might happen more frequently. I work in critical care so the needs of my patients are emergent. There are days I give a drug for an emergent intubation or seizure then I work backwards from administration of the order given by a doctor verbally as a patient is being intubated or seizing.

You know, placing the order in the computer for the medications after the fact. Cause, saving the life is first, right? Even in no emergent situations docs will often call out an order to you as they visit with the patient on daily rounds. Sometimes those orders sound a lot like general conversation. " I think he might benefit from 40 of lasix.' You should immediately follow-up with the question. 'Are you going to put in the order for lasix? ' They will tell you if they are; again use your 5 rights to get order facts straight. Put in the order while they are looking at you is the best thing.

Get in the habit of repeating and writing down those orders no matter how they are given to you. You absolutely must, must repeat the order to them and try to put it in the computer as you are repeating it to them. If at all possible ask for the ordering provider to put the order in themselves. Some will oblige, while others will look at you like you just asked them to walk backwards 10 miles while flying a kite. It will not take you long to sort out who is who here so don't stress about it. It goes without saying that if you do call a doc at home; prepare to add the order yourself. If you are unsure if they will enter it just ask them.

Third, take a deep breath and remember these are dynamic patients. They are not static so things are likely to change. That means that you should check your orders often. Sometimes just acknowledging this helps to alleviate your anxiety.

If the order changes it is not a signal you did something wrong. Patient orders are supposed to change as the patient is on the mend.

Fourth, be easy on yourself, sunshine. Within six months you will get to know the standard order sets and preferences of the docs that frequent your unit. You will also be in the habit of checking the order set at shift start and frequently throughout your day. They can change quickly and no one will tell you that they change, as I learned the hard way.

You will not get a courtesy call from Doctor Awesome to say, 'oh by the way, Nurse Awesome, I changed Mr. Smith's antibiotic to Zosyn since his Vancomycin level was so high so please do not give that 0900 vancomycin.' That vancomycin will not always be removed from the patients medication supply either. It is more likely to be that 2 hours later, once you have hung the Vancomycin; you see that the doctor changed the order. Rats!

Checking orders often not only keeps your patients safe it also takes out some of the rework and backtrack in your day. For example, maybe you pulled your meds for 10 am and one of those is Dilantin. You do 50 other things before you give that med. You sit down 20 minutes later to chart then see there is a new order for a level to be done before the dose you just gave. Ugh! Good to get in the habit of double checking the orders prior to med admin, it takes a second however; it will save you a lot of headache in the long run.

Sometimes there will be multiple doctors putting in orders. They do not always talk to one another before doing that. One doc wants to give ½ NS and the other says NS. Maybe the regular doc asks for a 150 ml/hour of NS to be given to the patient but the kidney doc has stated they want a KVO only drip going. Do not be afraid to speak up and ask questions. Do not just follow the orders if they make no sense to you. Most docs are happy to answer questions about why they are treating in a certain way.

If the order makes no sense do not carry out that order until you question it, please. We learned this firmly with drugs like beta-blockers, remember?

There were some strict rules about giving this medication. Don't give the drug if the SBP is <90 or the HR is <60, right? So let's say the doctor doesn't set a parameter in his order. In other words, he doesn't give you RULE to follow that says..If SBP=_____ or HR=_____then hold this order. Doctor Awesome still wants you to use your nursing judgment to hold the order if a SBP or HR is already low. If your patient has a low HR or SBP and you give him a beta blocker then call your physician and tell him that the patient is now profoundly hypotensive or bradycardic and ask for help correcting that prepare to get yelled at by that doctor. Just sayin..

Well, the same holds true for every medication. It also holds true for ever order. In other words, just because the doctor wrote the order for the patient to be out of bed for meals does not mean that you need to haul your patient with a systolic blood pressure of 65 who is also having trouble breathing out of the bed for lunch for the sake of following the order. Don't do this unless you are prepared to pick your passed-out patient off the floor and report the fall or work a code.

This is what I mean by using it as a guide but not a literal translation. Use your critical thinking skills first and be strong enough to say no if you need to protect the patient.(*Note to Self*-It is good practice to document anytime you deviated from an order and why somewhere in the chart.)

Communication is the key to safe + effective patient care.

For me , the biggest impediment to getting in a good flow with handling issues with doctors orders this first month really started and stopped within me. My own ego, my own fear, my own nerves.

Somehow I got myself all worked up about what it means to 'question' a doctor. Somehow I lost site of the fact that most docs really do depend on us to be the *most current* set of eyes on that patient. Did you hear that? Depend. On.

The doctor will see and assess the patient and write orders based on that assessment. What if the doc saw the patient at 0600 and you shift starts at 1900. What if that patients vitals or assessment data have changed in some manner. The doctor cannot see that information so he trusts that you will protect your mutual interest (the health and safety of your patient).

Seriously, it does not matter if you are on day 1 of your nursing career; docs actually depend on your current assessment of the patient. You are a team, right?

Taking a minute to let that sink in my nervous newbie brain changed everything. I flipped it from the 'questioning a doctor' place in mind that freaked me out to the 'protecting our mutual interest' place. This simple shift in my own thinking helped my nerves go-away.

If you find yourself nervous about talking to doctors when you have a question or need a new order stop and examine the reasons behind it.

Are you nervous because you are afraid they will ask you a question you do not have the answer for at that moment? Are you shaky because you lack confidence over all? Have you already decided in your head that you are going to get 'yelled' at so you are worked up over nothing? Is this the doctor everyone hates to call?

I work with a brain surgeon that no one likes to call. This doctor is brilliant and most days will leave detailed instructions in their orders. They round on the patient morning and night. The doc expects the nurse to look at the chart up front and see what might be needed for that patient, whether it is a pain med, sleeping pill or something to help them poop. They want you to ask when they are there and save the middle of the night calls for the BIG things like, 'our patient has seized' or 'our patient had put out 3000ml of urine in 2 hours', they will be cross if you wake them up to ask for Tylenol or Colace.

Come on, that might tick you off a little bit too, right? *(Note to Self*: this would be good info to pass to the next nurse.)

You will learn the docs that come to your unit quickly. Until then here are some simple fixes for calling the doctor jitters:

- Try to form your own opinions here and just let the experience happen before you decide that it will suck.
- You know more than you think. Remember when you learned all those 'standard doses' for medication in you pharm class? This is where you use them. If a doc calls out a verbal order for 15mg dose of a medication that is usually given in mcg then this is your chance to catch it.
- Review the chart, the current medications and the current vital signs before you call the doctor/before they round. Jotting down the latest and greatest labs at the start of every shift is always a good idea. Know the I/O's for your shift and the one before. What was already tried for this issue? Be able to tell them all these things will help them do their job and will gain

you confidence in your own ability and gain you credibility with the doctors at the same time.

- If you call them make sure you really need to call them. Ask a co-worker for their opinion if you are having trouble interpreting an order, first. It always helps to have a second set of eyes when you have trouble. Do it before you call Dr. Awesome.
- Stand up and speak up if something does not make sense. The more you practice articulating in the language of medicine the better you get and the more confident you become.

Foster the belief that docs actually want you to think for yourself and to ask questions. While they may gripe about it, they will appreciate it.

Look, physicians are not perfect and they know it, they want you to have their back. They are human and they do get stressed and sometimes crabby. Be okay with that fact...quickly or you will be a basket case.
As crabby as you think they may get with you, they DO expect you to advocate for the patient before you allow yourself to be scared/pushed around or otherwise fail to advocate for the patient because of their crabbiness.

All the professionals you work with will put you on equal footing with them when you start. It is amazing the way this happens but I have seen it over and over again. You are a colleague and they will show you respect. They will only start to question you when you give them reason to question you (unless they are a CV surgeon then they question everyone). The easy fix for this is to just take a minute to be thorough and think things out before you call. No sweat!

You worked hard to develop that nurse brain of yours so flaunt that bad boy. Use your critical thinking skills + question things that might not make sense; including doctor's orders.

Focus Point: You'll gain confidence in this area quickly. Your patient is depending on you to conquer your own fears in order to protect them. This is an area where we need to see your light shine. Talking to doctors will not be the hardest job you face....

Action Step: Ask for some clear guidelines about doctors' verbal orders and how they are entered in your state. Do it now before you do it wrong and get accused of practicing medicine.

Mantra Mojo: *I will stay committed to patient safety no matter how crazy the shift gets.*

Strong Work Today, Star shine!

You did a great job protecting your license today in the middle of all that craziness.

You were even able to tell the doctor no without making him feel horrible for asking you to do something he knows you should not be doing in the first place.

Way to consider everyone in the process.

You are a rock star..Don't forget it!

Love

Me

NEEDY PATIENTS + THEIR FAMILIES

Welcome to your shift. Your lunch is in the fridge, stethoscope around your neck and pens in your pocket. You've been briefed by the charge nurse and have your patient assignments in hand. You have even spent a bit of time in the patient chart so you have a handle on what kind of care you will need to provide. You are prepared to have an awesome shift.

As you walk around the corner, the nurse about to give you report is sitting with her bag on the desk, her head in her hands, tapping her feet. She looks up to greet you with an enthusiastic, "I am sooooo glad to see you!"

Your otherwise sunny disposition melts in one second because you know that the expression on her face can only mean one thing:

Caution, High-Maintenance Patient + Family Ahead.

No one wants to see this look. It can make 12 hours feel like 1200. It is especially bad if the nurse giving report spills a boatload of actual medical issues peppered in-between the rants about the level of crazy attached to your patient. Actual illness coupled with neediness make you work hard for your money. Period.

So take a breath before you brady-down and pass out. You just passed the NCLEX. You are tough stuff. A cray-cray patient and their family is something you can handle. All you need is a solid plan to navigate the shift without ending up in the nuthouse yourself.

First things first, cut yourself a bit of slack. After all, you're still trying to get your bearings on the floor, learning the unit management and what they expect you to 'take' from this population. Until you get a good feel for this it can be tough to know how firmly you can draw lines with these folks.

Gentleness with self, check!

Now, when you find yourself with one of these patients I want you to shout-'Yes! I am getting a crash course in communication!' Then, I want you to truly be grateful. Cause while 12 hours with these folks can feel like forever you will be so much smarter when shift is done. You really will feel like you have just taken a Tony Robbins crash course, seriously.
There will be several types of crazy-folk that come into Smiley General for help. The...I have no real medical reason for the crazies but I am neurotic and needy and scared, folks and the honest-to-goodness demented, bipolar, I am not in my right mind' patients.

There is a wide variation on these 2 themes. Usually they fall somewhere in-between. You can't quite be mad at them but they can irritate you to no end trying to figure out how to get them to calm down.

This chapter focuses on those humans that are just plain old needy and scared. *(Note to Self*: dementia is a whole different animal.)

School was not realistic in the way we cared for these folks. As a student nurse, I knew I did not HAVE to deal with 100 shades of crazy behavior, I did not have to take verbal beatings, I knew that afternoon post conference was always at 4pm and I did not have to come back the next day to do it all over again.

Needless to say when I got my first high maintenance patient and had to attend to them for a full 12 hour shift I left the floor totally beat. I felt a little more like a babysitter than a nurse and it pissed me off to waste an entire shift. This is not what I spent years buried in a textbook for at all! It was all about getting in the head space of another human in order to ratchet them down from a 20 to somewhere around a 5 on the anxiety scale. Instead of exercising my technical skills it was all about distraction, negotiation and patience.

What tools do you have to help keep these folks from losing their shit through the shift while keeping a handle on your own? Take a breath, and know that you started gathering these tools long before you ever came into a nursing program. You just need to recall where you put them and learn how to focus them.

Let's do a little free-flow writing about how you might handle some crazy patient behavior. What will you do if they are on the call bell non-stop?

What if their demands are unreasonable? What if they scream in pain every time you touch them and even when you do not touch them?

What if their pain level never comes below 10? What if the crazy person is the family? Got some ideas??

Here are the tools that I used to help myself adjust to these types of shifts:

1st tool: Start your shift with a blank slate!

Good GAWD, this is a powerful tool. Think of it. No preconceived notions in your head at all about the patient or the shift. What?!

Yep, you gotta do it. Level these folks in your head. What on earth does that mean? Well, I mean, you have to let go of any preconceived notions or judgment of them. Let go of the previous nurse's view of them.

You have no clue what is really making them act this way and you will not figure that out in 12 hours so don't try.

Just treat them as humans, you know? Be kind for goodness sakes!

While you can't get deep into their head it is actually pretty easy to understand what they need. Empathy can go a long way to bridge the gap between you.

If all else fails apply the Golden Rule liberally.

2nd tool: Find the story behind their story

Ask yourself, what is this patient really trying to tell you?

They are afraid. They are in pain. Their needs are not being met. They have no control. They are having withdrawal from that 'one' glass of wine per night they told you about. They need a Xanax.

All of the above really but most importantly, they are telling you that they feel scared and that they do not trust that you will be able to keep them safe. That is a huge bummer, huh?

If it is the family that has a bit of the 'cray-cray' then they are feeling the same.

Imagine if you were stuck in a strange place with strange people and felt like you might die. Suck-Central and not a good feeling, huh?

Imagine if your loved one were in that position and you had to trust in those caring for the person most important to you in the entire world. Still not a good feeling, huh?

Ah, the power of empathy~

This is one of the big 'whys' behind obnoxious patient behavior.

We have all felt it at some point in our shift. They ring the call bell constantly to know that you notice what is going on with them, that you are paying attention. They need you close in case they need saving. They are asking for assurance that you care about them, that you will not let them die.

The best action from you is to relieve the uncertainty they are feeling. Tell them the plan for their care for that shift, tell how often you will check on them, tell them the side effects they may feel from the meds you give them, tell them the things that they MUST call you for and then show them how to use the call bell plus, reassure them that you will respond promptly. Then follow through with your plan + respond promptly.

A couple of hours into the shift, when you have done exactly what you told them you would do, you usually will see these patients morph into pleasant and not so stressed humans. Some people will still treat the call bell like concierge service; most will calm down with some conscientious practice.

Remove their uncertainty and they have no need for drama.

Other times the folks that sit on the call bell are telling us:
> They have uncontrolled anxiety,
> They are angry that they let their health get to this place
> They are in information overload or need it in understandable terms
> They feel out of control + they do not trust us

I get my share of the families you get warned about. I don't mind all that much in fact, I like the challenge of figuring out what will calm them and then doing it.

Most of the time, spending a bit of time with them up front communicates that you care enough about them and their loved one that they will loosen up the death grip they have on your time.

There are folks that are actually dealing with clinical issues only a psychiatrist can address. Don't beat yourself up for not being able to calm them and just hold on for your shift.

3rd tool: Be.Here.Now.

Giving them your full presence: Smile at them and mean it. Tell them you appreciate being allowed to care for them. Let them know you 'know' being sick is hard.

Case in Point:

I had a patient my first month on my own that was what you might call a 'piece of work'. This person was sick, cranky, had escaped death more than once in the last year and was an expert at working the call bell. This was not the patient I wanted to be with all shift. I admit the first time I got this assignment that I was bit apprehensive about the whole thing. If the unit 'lore' was true it would be a miserable 12 hours.

Instead of getting sucked into what someone else told me would happen I projected a few good thoughts in front of me and went confidently into the room at shift change with the voice of Ivan Drago in my head: ' I will break you' .

The lore was pretty spot on. Within 2 hours between the tech, me and other nurses, someone had been in the room 13 times.

This not an exaggeration.

Having no clue what was 'really' going on with the patient I tucked my other patient in and went into the room of call-bell abuser patient and sat down. Communication was made tough by some medical conditions however; I can be creative when needed.

So I got creative, I watched TV, I bathed them and made them help me, I fluffed pillows, I shared stories about my kids and my pets, I told jokes.

At the end of almost 2 hours the patient was smiling. Holy dinger, all that person needed was my full presence. Making that effort proved that I cared for them and about them and that somehow magically gave them a sense that I would not let them die that shift. I left the room telling the patient I would be back in one hour to check on them and followed through on that commitment. My shifts with them after this day were fairly peaceful and without the abuse of a call light system.

Never underestimate the power of your presence.

You are a force of nature, you!

4th tool: Invite Trust

Never underestimate your importance in their healing. You are only with them for 12 hours however; your attitude and your full presence can set them up for some incredible healing that continues long after you are gone. It can change the way they look at their disease and their role in it. It can set them up to work as a partner with the healthcare system instead of against it. The only way this happens is if you work hard to build trust. Some ways to accelerate trust:

- o Personalize your patient. That is, remember they are a person not a room number. We get kind of calloused to things quickly. In part, that is needed for survival; especially in some of the areas of critical care. Room numbers are not people!
- o Give them the chance to ask your questions at the start of the shift, explain to them what the shift is going to be like for them, tell them what the plans are(include lab testing/xray, OOB times, baths or other hygiene),
- o Never give a med to a conscious and mentally present patient without telling them what you are giving them and why, tell them if there is a change they could make in their lifestyle that may result in no longer needing the med one day
- o Never leave the room without asking them if there is something else they need to be more comfy before you leave. Give them an estimate on when you will be back. Then do it, building trust doesn't take long and neither does destroying it
- o Be proactive-You received a good bit of intel from the nurse that gave you report. The statement, 'Your other nurse told me you were concerned about_____' works wonders! It tells them they were important enough to pass on at shift change.

I found it by accident in the middle of a shift with a super-needy daughter whose parent was three days post-op and couldn't seem to move out of the ICU. After she had laid on her parents call bell for about two hours solid I finally asked her what she was truly nervous about. Aside from the obvious fear of death, she was worried that sweating meant they were spiking a temperature and that we were doing nothing about it because fever meant infection and infection meant death. I explained to her that we were checking temp frequently and thought this would calm her however; no sooner than I walked out of the room than she was on the call bell again in order to show me the beads of sweat on her loved ones forehead. It was in a moment of desperation bordering on facetious that I handed her the thermometer and showed her how to use it along with a piece of paper with half hour increments written across the top. I told her I was super-busy and that if she could help me take the temp every 30 minutes and write it down that it would help me a lot. I explained how a temp of less than 100.1 was acceptable and did not need medication and gushed about how much I appreciated the effort on their part. I never expected it to settle her emotions and calm her nerves. Thankfully, it did.

I still use the temperature trick a lot when family members need to feel in control of something. It doesn't hurt me or my patient one single bit to have the family checking it and it certainly gives them a sense that they did something to help. I also get the family to help me with the pain scale or with positioning arms and legs (provided there are no limitations here) to help them feel like they are doing something productive for the person they love.

6th tool: Empathy Please

Learn a bunch of non-religious, non judgmental, supportive things to say to someone in pain.

- I know I can't fix this for you. Let's see what we can do to make it better though.
- I know the doctor has explained things however; if you still have questions I am here to help.
- I cannot imagine how you must feel. I want you to know your feelings matter to me.
- I will work hard to provide you excellent care.
- This must feel really frustrating for you. I am sorry, how can I help?
- You look well today, tell me though, how are you feeling?

Expressing some interest in them other than medication administration works wonders to calm them down.

If all else fails just try to realize up front that people do stupid things when they are sick and scared. Logical, level-headed, productive members of society become your worst nightmare when they are down. This is just one of those traits that humans can have a hard time getting away from it seems. Not everyone, of course, but damn, you are going to see some uber-smart people acting odd.

Another case in Point:

I had a patient's husband insist on taking off his wife's BIPAP to allow her to eat. He was an engineer, he was not without intelligence yet over + over he would remove it, she would swallow and her O2 alarms would go nuts and he would ring the call bell frantically. The machines coupled with her graying pallor made him nuts and the number flashing on the screen coupled with the wife's widening eyes flung him totally over the edge into anxiety town; yet he kept doing it. To him, not feeding her was the same as killing her; it is that way for lots of folks. I calmly explained the reason for the BIPAP and added a line or two about the need for oxygen usurping the need for food and being in an ICU not at home so the choices change. I also explained to him that his actions were making things worse for his beloved; not better. He stopped removing the BIPAP. Turns out when I asked her if she was hungry she shook her head no anyway. She had been eating so he would feel like he was doing something to help her heal. Funny how they were just loving each other, huh?

I had to set some firm rules with him. I tried to meet his need to feel like he was contributing to his healing for his loved one while providing a safe space for the patient to heal in by giving him another task. He actually appreciated that I set some rules for him that day and taught him how to care for her in a way he would need when they went home from the hospital.

It is important to set boundaries for your patients and their families. You are in control here.

Never forget that your primary objective is to keep the patient safe. This guiding principle can make it easier to draw lines with tough families and knowing you're most concerned about keeping their loved one safe, even when you are drawing lines for them not to cross, will give comfort to those freaked out people. Do not be afraid to say exactly that to your family or patient. 'My first job is to keep you safe so you cannot do_____.'

Patients can go through some fairly large extremes in emotion while hospitalized. I would say that most of the time the emotions are legit.

That said though, the world tolerates people acting like assholes and so sometimes you are going to have a patient that just chooses to be a handful. I try to label that behavior 'scared' before I label it 'asshole'. Not because it helps them but because it helps me not to be pissy with them as I care for them for 12 hours by believing they are afraid.

After all, none of us really knows what happens next, right?

Learning how to negotiate care with people who are stressed takes time so if you have a rough go of it the first few times you take care of one of these folks don't sweat it, please. You will learn and you will develop your own style of communication with your patients. It will be based off those non-negotiable items you have decided to bring into your practice.

Everyone has the potential to be less than cooperative, needy or downright neurotic. Keep these things in your tool kit cause at some point you are going to land smack in the middle of crazy town with a patient. They will make for smoother sailing through the shift.

People want to trust you. If they have been dismissed by other nursing staff then it is harder to gain that trust.

You will need to turn your compassion on high for these peeps.
You will need to accept that they will be unreasonable and that it will take a minute to gain their trust. You also need to understand that once you gain their trust you will not have any more issues from them. At least 90% of the time.

It can be hard to have empathy when the person doing the complaining actually caused the illness themselves. You know the diabetic that was told years ago to check his blood sugar and use insulin but refused to do that at all. Or the 400 lb guy that just had a CABG complaining about the procedure or pain associated with it. As you dig down deep to find your empathy you start to get into the art of our craft rather than just the science.

I always take the time to say something positive to every person I speak with each night.

Phrases that start with I appreciate you when... I respect that you... I never thought of doing it like this... I admire your experience... Thank you for sharing...

These are more than just for your peer group of nurses.

A few months are not enough time to get good at dealing with the cray-cray bunch.

It is reasonable to ask yourself to learn to recognize the behavior patterns of a frightened person in 30 days. It is reasonable to ask yourself to create some soothing statements for different types of patients and it is reasonable to expect yourself to exercise empathy and patience. Use that in equal doses for you and the patient + family.

It is not reasonable to think you will maintain your composure 100% of the time or that you will not be ticked off by these folks or pushed to the edge of your niceness. I have seen even the most seasoned person lose their cool with a high maintenance person at hour 11.

It will help if you can look to the family as an extension of your patient. While your primary concern is the patient in the bed the whole lot of them has needs to meet.

The patient will feel it if you go into the room with your defensive posture all up in their grill.

They will feel that you do not want to be there. Use your power for good here and it will change your shift. If you need to go collect yourself for a minute by all means do so just do not set yourself up for failure by carrying the chip from the old nurses shoulder into the room on your own.

When all else fails repeat in your mind over and over; Needy patients need my time, needy patient need my time...

Free style some ways to deal with non-productive patient behavior. How will you know when you need a time-out from that patient?

Focus Point: Needy patient are almost always scared humans.

Action Step: Make extra time for at least one needy patient this week. See if your time can change their mindset of fear

Mantra Mojo: *I am kind and loving at all times*

TAKE 5...

The 5 most moving + surprising things you learn quickly that no amount of schooling can teach...

You can get a patient to tell you almost anything with a popsicles+ a pillow flip. Both are magic portals to soulful conversation

People want to trust you with their life

Very few people feel empowered to make life-changing choices in their own life

Every day + every patient can change you for the better; if you allow it

There are worse things than death

IF ALL ELSE FAILS

This chapter is nothing new.

You learned these concepts in your first semester of school.

Don't go thinkin that just because you are all 'grown-up' now that you won't need them anymore. Quite the contrary; now you will use them more than ever!

The core components of your nursing practice are your friend.

They will keep your patient safe and keep your license safe as well.

I looked to these as floaties on the days when I was drowning in the sea of newness to keep myself a float and I carried them in my pocket on an index card along with my major action for major events for the first 2 months on the job

That might sound truly pathetic. It really gave me HUGE peace of mind to know that I was not going to have to remember everything in a crisis so for me, this small action was worth looking pathetic over.

Knowing they were there if needed helped me 'feel' more like a nurse even when I left the shift exhausted. You can expand this list to your own. Just ask yourself, what information/idea/med knowledge/procedure steps would keep you a float?

Psst..Don't forget to...

Wash your hands..a lot!
Use 2 patient identifiers
Check room safety-Bag mask nearby, O2 setup, bed in lowest position, wheels locked, call bell in reach

Use ABC's, Maslow's / Erickson's to prioritize patient care
Scan your medications-look for parameters to give that the doc sets
Look up the med if you don't know about it before you give it-don't forget to teach them about it
Explain the side effects to the patient so they can report the abnormal to you
Drugs like Digoxin, dilantin and vancomycin should trigger in your head..LABS..as in do I need to draw them before I give this dose
Act with integrity in all you do
Have Compassion and treat people the way you want to be treated
Know Normal Vitals/Know Normal Labs/O2 use basics
Positioning-helping out of bed
Precautions/Isolation needs

Now, for something a little less pathetic, let's see if we can prepare for your First Code. You walk into the room of your nice little 50 year old laparoscopic cholecystectomy. She is face down on the floor, what do you do?

Go...quickly

1. Attempt to arouse your patient by calling their name and using some pain
2. If not responsive then check for pulse in two locations
3. If no pulse follow your procedure for calling a code(button on the wall/bed/phone)
4. Start CPR. Do not go running out of the room to get the crash cart. Start CPR. I work in an ICU so I can call for help and get 4 people there in about a second. This is one of those luxuries you don't get on the floor. Either way, you have to take control.
5. The next thing you need to do is start to tell people what you need from them. Do not be afraid to take control of your patient and this space you are in with them at this moment just because you have less experience of your space and your code. The first

thing out of your mouth should be "I need the crash cart". If there is family present ask them to please step outside, explaining that there will be a lot of activity going on around their loved one.

6. As soon as a doc arrives start to tell him the background on the patient and what happened preceding this event. Do not wait for them to ask you. Speak up and do it quickly.

7. Once the doc gets there they will take over directing people around. By the time the crash cart gets there you will have some help. A lot of help and probably at least one doctor from ICU or ED to run things for you, thankfully...

We had a code day at my school. This is a skills lab where you go through several scenarios and walk through the steps above over and over again. This repetition serves to root the sequence of steps in your brain. The first time you have to go through a code on one of your patients you will probably forget at least half of them.

So reduce it down to the needed parts in your noggin.

Airway, breathing and circulation; check.

The first 2 months I was a nurse I did the code drill in my head every day on the way into work. As soon as I actually got into the patient room I scouted out the stool, made sure I could work the bed and double-checked for the presence of the ambu bag. Every shift and every patient without fail. That is still part of my safety check every shift.

Run through it in your head every day until you get the hang of it. When it feels second nature to you then run through it some more. You will silently be losing your shit the first day you actually have to run a code.

Look for something that has to be done. If no one is recording do that, if no one has gotten the crash cart, do that. You will be thankful as hell when the rest of the team arrives and someone takes over. Seriously.

If you need to, as soon as a more experienced nurse comes in let them take over but tell them that you need them to take over. Do not just assume they will do it because they have experience.. No one will look down on you for doing this, they know they have experience and you do not. They were new once too. Differ to the brain-trusts that have been there forever. As you do that though, study exactly what they do to the extent possible in the crisis. Jot it down and ask them questions about why they made the choices they made when they did a little later when you have some time. Next time you will be more empowered to reach half their brain size

Come back to this page often and jot down what you see in your specific unit are those areas that you need to know that you know that you know them....That is what this extra space is for..doodles are okay too!

Meanwhile back at stately Wayne Manor, there is another, less talked about, aspect of the code.

DEATH

Not something that most of us want to talk about really.

It is important for you to have worked out your own views on death, what you think happens to you after death, do you have a soul and all that before you start nursing for real.

This is important because you are going to see a lot of death. It is a super-charged thing+ emotions run high even if you did not know the decedent well. Having a firm root in your own belief system will keep you from getting knocked over when you have to deal with other peoples difficulties surrounding dying family members. Watching another human take their last breath while you are in charge of keeping them alive is tough stuff.

An equally important thing to get quick is a softness within you about how other people come to the moment of death and how families cope with it. I have seen grown people in their 60's hysterically begging a doc to keep their 92 year old parent alive. I have watched many people die slow and painful (at least what I believe is painful) because no one worked it out ahead of time. It will cause you some internal conflict if you do not take some time and examine how you feel about keeping someone alive with 'all medical means'.

Truth is, as morally hard as it is, you have to arrive at the place where you 'know' it is not your call to make, it's only the patient and the family that get to decide when 'enough is enough'. The quicker you can get to a place of non-judgmental detachment about it the better it is for everyone involved. Don't expect any certain behavior just let the family have whatever expression of grief they need to release that loved one. As long as it takes.

When I first started nursing, I seriously wanted to pummel any family that let a PEG tube and tracheotomy happen on a family member past the age of 85; particularly if that patient already had dementia or some sort of debilitation that made their quality of life horrible. After wrestling with it a lot I can honestly say that only part of the time do I manage to stay in a detached place about it. It is super-hard for me to watch people suffer when families leave them alone in the hospital. I have lost a lot of sleep about it. I truly love other humans and it is inhumane. It sends my heart into full tilt boogie. That said, it is not my call to make really, ever, it is not always easy to keep my mouth shut about it. I work on this daily in order to support all involved without feeling like I am contributing to the suffering of the patient.

As harsh as it sounds when I find myself in these spots I just say silently to myself, 'not my circus, not my monkeys' to flip things in my brain to the place I know that I am not in charge. I don't use that statement to insinuate that death is funny at all, it just triggers my brain to stop obsessing about it and helps me know the only thing I am charged to do is keep them alive for 12 hours; regardless of any other factor.

Have you had a patient code and die on you yet in your clinical rotations? A code is an all out effort to thwart the angel of death and it sucks to lose a patient this way. Invariably you will question something you did and think that you 'could have' done something to prevent the death.

It doesn't matter what the situation is you are going to wonder if there was something that you could have done to prevent this death. It doesn't matter what condition the patient was in when they got to you. It does not matter if this is a 95 year old with pneumonia that is DNR that you watch pass on comfort care.

There will be this piece of you that is human that says, 'I should have done more'.

Humans are like this with each other.

So look, you have to remember that we all die, right? Some people way before we think they should and some way after we think they should. We are not in control. Any other thoughts are just our own filter on top of the situation. This is where your belief system comes into play. Regardless of the particular brand of 'The Creator' you favor, we know that we all physically end one day. Not one of the world's religions has been able to escape that, prevent it or what-have-you. We end.

To be totally blunt here, the fact of it is that the person you are coding is most likely already dead when we come upon the code, right? That is how we know we need to do CPR, unstable or missing vitals signal to us that we need to start attempting to restore those vitals and save their life. With no intervention they would be dead.

Sometimes you bring them back to life and sometimes not. The thing is that you are in control of 'some' things. How quickly you react, how effective your compressions are etc, BUT ultimately you are not in control. Unless you have watched them going downhill for hours and can intervene pre-code, there is no magic eraser big enough to wash away death.

I spent a lot of time perplexed after my first patient death. We spent tons of time in nursing school learning about diseases that many of us will not even experience in our entire career and hardly any time learning about death; the one thing we will **all** experience in our career and life.

Sure we learned about the physical process of dying and

what vitals do and what we can expect to see when someone dies. We talked about post-mortem care and talking with families and all.

What I mean is that we did not actually talk about what you do with what you *feel* or the emotions that pop up when a death occurs.

There seems to be this odd expectation that you should know how to deal with death simply because you are human and will die one day yourself.
The first time you lose a patient it will suck worse than any NCLEX question or all night care plan session ever could. The first time that you have to look at a loved one and explain how Me-Maw crumped after you convinced them to go home and sleep; you will have difficulty with words. It is not easy however; with some work you can become an incredible facilitator of that transition to the next place. Wherever you believe it is we go.

If you don't have a good support system for when that happens (and it will) it might lead to a place where you don't process your feelings, you stuff them, you avoid them and then it turns into PTSD; you don't want this to happen.

So be an awesome nurse, already. Know this is going to happen and make a plan for gosh sakes. Investigating your options before you are dealing with it may be the best path for some of you that tend to OCD over things. Chaplains, unit support groups, a more experienced nurse buddy? Any of this will help.

Planned death or withdrawal of care is of course, a different matter which requires a different level of participation from you. When the death is planned then the best thing you can do is actively participate with the patient and the family to the extent the family and patient need. It is an extreme honor to get to be with someone when they take their last breath. We need help being born and sometimes we need help dying. If you can get your head in the right space about it and view yourself as a midwife to the next part of the human adventure it will help a lot. Viewing my role as an active participant in ushering them to the other side is sometimes the only thing that keeps me okay with how much death happens in ICU.

At some point in the process of dying your patient shifts from the one that occupies the bed and becomes the family. They don't always say it however; usually they are looking to you to help them make sense of what is going on. Medical sense, as in tell them what to expect next, as well as from an emotional standpoint.

You do not need to give them the textbook definitions of mottling or point out the Cheyne-Stokes breathing to them. They just need to know what to expect. If you have ever had a family member in hospice you know what this is like. Damn it is painful to sit there and wonder if every breath they take will be the last. Most families need to hear that the choice they made was the best. Lots of times there is not much you can say. Your presence is just as powerful as words.

Yes, expected death is tough although somewhat easier.

Here are some tips that might help:

Make your presence known to them and let them know you are just a voice away.

Explain to the family what you are doing when you are discontinuing care and starting comfort care only. Tell them you have stopped supporting breathing + blood pressure and that doing this allows a natural death. Make sure you know that you are not speeding up the dying process, just providing supportive care. Many, many people believe that morphine given is to make the death 'faster'. This is far from true. It simply helps the difficulty with breathing and the pain that can be associated with some disease states. Explain until the family feels safe that this will make breathing easier and calm any pain but that will not hasten death. (NTS-This is one of those areas family members carry guilt around once the loved one is gone.)

Do your best to provide the facts, without any religious interpretation by you, so that they have that solid base of knowledge for a few months down the road when they start their grieving process. It will help them to know 'everything' was done for their loved one. Offer to get them a chaplain if needed.

Set up the room before they get there. Get tissues, get extra chairs, turn down the lights if the bright ones are on and clean up the room.
Ask them what they need from you. Some people want you right there and others want you to leave them alone. Please, make sure to turn the damn monitors off. If there is a large family presence I feel a little like the door greeter at church. If the death is not expected then you may all just muddle through it together, tears and all.

Once everything is done you will need time to process what you just witnessed and participated in, too. We all do that differently. I always make sure that I find a minute with the patient while providing care at end of life to lean over into their ear and let them know; they mattered, I am thankful for knowing and caring for them, they will be missed, and in some way I thank them for the work they did while on the earth. I let them know they will not be forgotten and then post death I put my hand on their head and their heart and thank them again and tell them to have safe travels.

You will develop your own way to cope. I feel like my actions honor the person's spirit. That may just be a pile of crap I tell myself however; it helps me.

It will matter if you have taken care of this person a long time. A hospice worker will likely have more to grieve at the loss of a patient than a nurse in the emergency department that never actually spoke with a coding patient.

There is not a wrong or right answer when it comes to how you handle death. You could get some training if you feel it is needed. I did this because I knew it would help me cope. It is highly likely that experience will be the best teacher though. Your hospital offers some type of chaplain service for families and it is there for you as well. Do not be afraid to use it. Debrief with other nurses, talk to your floor manager. Sometimes the best thing for you is to talk about how you feel so that you realize you are not alone. You get better at knowing your role, especially if the death is planned and you get faster at assimilating what just happened, letting it go and moving forward. That is only because you gather more tools to help you as you have more experience though, not because it gets easier.

Some death will seem senseless and tragic while other times death may be seen as a welcome relief from a long term condition in which the patient suffered a lot. Either way, it still hurts you when it happens. You hang your head for a moment, say a prayer and move forward. Reach out for support when you need it.

One of the most difficult yet sacred things about the work we do is the presence of death.

Focus Point: Everyone comes at death with a different back story. Remaining neutral like Switzerland is the best stance to take

Action Step: Explore your feelings about death. Do you have good coping and support mechanisms in place?

Mantra Mojo: *Death happens for us all. I am open to being a loving support for my patients and their families through that process*

PTSD IN NURSES

I cannot tell you the number of sideways looks I got when I first mentioned post traumatic stress to an experienced nurse. I knew there was no way in heck that I was the only nurse having a problem digesting all the suffering I was witnessing on the daily.

It was surely not ever on my radar of 'possible' complications to being a nurse so I reckoned it was not on the radar of others either.

I was about a month into my first job as a nurse when I first started thinking 'something is not right' in the land of milk and honey (aka nursing). While I couldn't quite put my finger on it, this 'thing' that I was feeling and seeing, it was totally different than the image I had spent the last 20+ years conjuring in my mind.

The happy big-hearted healers I imagined, well, mostly they were not present on my unit. No one was cruel to patients; they just were not overtly supportive either. I remember one night I was waiting for our pre-shift circle up time. Fellow nurses were trickling in the room. Everyone was cranky. I said hello, and smiled as I always do and not one of those people smiled back at me. Most everyone had something negative to say when I told them I was 'awesome'. Most of them rolled their eyes and laughed like they didn't believe my 'awesome' stance. As a new nurse I could not imagine what on earth was making these humans so miserable. (**NTS**: do not stop being happy cause others are not happy)

Here I was, happy to be involved in this noble profession. Finally, after so much sacrifice and study I 'got to be' a nurse. This is truly the way I viewed it, as a blessing, a privilege, an honor. I had spent a lot of time daydreaming about what nursing would be like; I conjured many images in my head about my career in nursing and what that would be like each day.

Hard work, self sacrifice, blood, humanity exposed to its core, some suffering and tears, a lot of connection to other humans and a helluvalot of love being exchanged. This pissed off at the world 'thing' I was seeing was truly throwing me for a loop
It was not part of my imaginings.

I checked with my nursing school posse and figured out that it was not just me or my hospital or my unit that was getting hit by the grumpies. It seemed to be everywhere and it seemed to be in all kinds of units. Labor & Delivery, Rehab, Skilled Nursing, Geri-Psych, ICU and Med/Surg; everyone shared similar stories.

Not many of the long-timers were happy. Even some of the people I graduated with were questioning their career change choice already. By month 6, I counted myself in that group.

My thoughts of creating a better way to support nurses were born during my first clinical of my first semester of nursing school. As expected, I witnessed extreme suffering however; I experienced something unexpected that changed my view of nursing altogether.

I shadowed a nurse with 10 years on me and witnessed her as she treated my patient so cold and impatiently that it literally made me cry. Her actions were so harsh I felt she had forgotten that her patient was a human being. It was a traumatic event for me.

I went home believing I had made a terrible mistake leaving

my job in the corporate world. I stayed in school but never forgot what I saw that day. From there forward, I purposefully watched how nurses treated patients and as school progressed I saw this same behavior; a lot. Yes, there were awesome examples of caring + compassionate nurses. There were an equal number that showed a callousness + frustration that I wanted nothing to do with personally.

I quickly came to believe that these nurses were brought into my life to help me craft my practice. To teach me what kind of nurse I did not want to be when I 'grew up'. I viewed the nurses as broken; burnt out, ready to retire. Sometimes I just classed them as plain old mean. I was convinced I would never become them.

I asked each of my preceptors how I could guard against one day becoming that nurse from my first semester. They gladly shared their own career transitions and most of them chuckled at my 'idea' that nurses could be in a harsh and over-demanding system without being eventually changed by that system.

Most of them said there was no way to 'avoid' it.

Their thoughts made me begin to notice the way the system treated nurses. I viewed the situation with a different set of eyes. It was possible for me to become the same as those nurses who I thought were so cruel. I understood that despite any amount of caring I may want to give my patients that I could become indifferent to the needs of my patients If I was not taking care of my own needs. I even saw the cruel behavior of that nurse from my first clinical day in a different way. It was not all her that was broken it was the system that supported her that was cracked.

By and large, nurses are dedicated and caring people who

view their work and their patients with the utmost importance. We are proud of the profession and enjoy the contribution we are making to the world. No matter how grumpy we appear we love our patients.

As a brand new nurse you are going to notice first and foremost that we are asked to perform at an unrealistic level daily. We are asked to speed through the day to get to charting that is 'required' from one governing body while complying with rules and regulations laid out by another governing body(who does not talk to the first one) under direction from still another group, all while providing excellent patient-centered-customer-service-oriented care deemed important by yet another entity altogether; our employer. The customer service bend is quickly teaching patients that they can get what they want when they want. This adds to the workload and frustration level and as a new nurse it is tough to know how to negotiate it.

We are told under penalty of law that we cannot practice 'medicine' yet simultaneously asked to be the second set of eyes for the physician by providing details on what we deem 'medically' important.

We are assumed to be an expert on pharmacology and the effects that multiple drugs will cause with the vast knowledge that one small semester of focused pharmacology in nursing school provides.

We are asked to teach and to adapt teaching styles to fit our individual patient with no formal teacher's certification.

We witness death in one room then gracefully enter another to calm down the self-centered patient who is angry the unit is too noisy when all we want to do is tell them they are more blessed than the guy next door to them.

We are counselors and project managers with no degrees in these fields who are expected to have the correct thing to say in multiple stressful situations and to be organized and efficient as if we did have those degrees.

We are expected to provide safe care for multiple sick patients that could become critically ill at any moment and families that could escalate as the patient does; with no formal time or crisis management training.

All of this is hard to digest, process, let go of..whatever you call it.

Many of us can suffer from PTSD-like affects without having ever stepped into a war zone.
So what I saw as a cranky and bitter nurse in my first semester was transformed. She was a product of the system detailed above. She was not the issue she was the result of no one addressing the issues within the system that had changed her entire way of being.

The gaps between the corporate hospital structures, government expectations and the reality of human limitations being reached actually produced a nurse who knew she faced a set of damn near impossible goals before she ever started the day, which in turn create a nurse with an over-full cup before they ever took care of a single patient.

Please be on the lookout for this within yourself. No matter how positive and sunny your disposition now. Eventually, your cup will get overfull. You must look for it so you can correct it.

I was not looking for PTSD. I mean, to me it was all about war and serious trauma/sexual assault victims and the like. Not once at work did I see a picture that even remotely resembled my idea of post traumatic stress disorder (PTSD for short). I have an uncle that served in Vietnam; I am friends with several Gulf War Vets. I have sat with single moms who were victims of some damn crazy events. My husband suffers from it because he was hit by a car while riding his bike. These are the pictures I held of PTSD and the only ones I imagine would benefit from PTSD assistance.

So count that as another place that I was wrong. PTSD can happen to damn near anyone; including nurses.

You have to find some support for these first months in practice. An internet board, a group, a life coach, a nurse buddy or whatever fits your style; finding a way to commiserate with like-minded folks and some way to reframe what you are going through is a must for your mental health.

Home support systems mean well. It is just that there are very few partners or family members that can empathize with you when you release the stress of watching 2 patients die, discharging another and getting 2 new patients in the same shift...very few unless they are also nurses. There is so much back-story that has to be told before you can even get to the meat of things that there is just no point.

Nurse-to-nurse support follows a bitch and moan type outlet more than a constructive; here is what can happen to turn this into good, place of support.

Instead of just listening to the vent/rage cycle we have to start listening to each other's hardship and then reflecting back the best parts of each other that may have gotten lost in the shuffle rather than bitching right along with our co-worker. We have to start helping each other recreate all the suffering so we can release it and move on.

There is room for us to change this within our profession and I think we can get to the heart of things together more quickly.

We also need to remove the stigma attached to being stressed.

I think it has to be okay to talk about how death affects you.

It has to be okay that watching the suffering of someone can harm you just as much as a death did.

It has to be okay that we feel and express that we feel used, overworked and uncared for by the fine folks of Smiley General.

It has to be okay to not be so strong that we know how to do everything already and ask for help.

It has to be okay to show vulnerability with each other.
It has to be okay to say, 'Holy crap, I am so overwhelmed I don't know how to get past it!'

None of those things are okay now.

Sure, on the surface it appears like it is fine for us to be less than super-people 24/7. Ask some nurses though, in private, without the fear of being tattled on to management or being labeled difficult and see how that answer changes.

Positive support should be a non-negotiable item.

Right now, the systems we inhabit looks at us like robots of some sort. In many cases our systems penalizes the person that asked for help. They are quick to note that a nurse is producing poor survey scores but not as quick to offer help to get to the bottom of why she is producing those poor scores.

My hope is that we can change that eventually.

Focus Point: PTSD is one of the pitfalls of our profession. Remain insightful about your feelings and attitudes and take action if you begin to feel overwhelmed.

Action Step: Learn the signs and symptoms of PTSD

Mantra Mojo: *I am in the flow of life. I accept change with ease and release any sadness I see*

In the meantime, y'all PTSD looks different in everyone. Here are some basics signs it might be happening for you.

PTSD Signs + Symptoms
- Depression
- Anxiety
- Unexplained Fear or hesitancy while performing familiar tasks
- Feelings of guilt
- Substance abuse or increase in use
- Problems with sleep, nightmares
- Problems with outbursts of tears or anger
- Sweating or shaking for unknown reasons
- Dizziness, appetite changes, headaches, chest pain
- Detachment from life or isolating yourself

You can do your part to facilitate this change by recognizing the symptoms of PTSD so that you can offer help to your peers, perhaps yourself, if you see them happening.

You can further help by taking a personal stand and

becoming one of those nurses that help your peer group remember they are awesome, that reflects the good qualities about their nursing practice and that helps your buddies recreate it, laugh it off or otherwise let it go. Please.

There are many resources on the web that can help with this issue. Your biggest challenge is to recognize it before it starts to govern your life and then find a constructive way to let go of the feelings, emotions and stress causing the issues.

If you really want to help change things, next time you are asked to be on a shared governance committee ask if you can start one about PTSD in your unit.

So wow Nurse Awesome–

You never expected it to be a good thing that you are coming at this career later in life, huh?

Put your hand in the air⋯woot woot!

The confidence you show your patients makes them much more comfy with the care you are providing. Funny that they all assume you have been a nurse forever. Thanks, grey hair!

And you were worried that your age would hurt you, ha!

You are a gorgeous force of nature + truly blessed to have the open soul you do, you are a wise-one disguised as a nurse.

Share from your heart and know this is all you ever have to do.

Don't forget to dance–

Me

2ND CAREER CHALLENGES

I chose to become a nurse when I was 23 and I finally graduated when I was 45; quite the seasoned vet when it came to the business of life I guess. Nursing, not so much.

There were some luxuries my age afforded that my younger counterparts simply could not find. I was calm under pressure, had the ability to let go of stress, had established the priorities in my life, my finances were in order and of course; I had an age-related confidence in unknown situations that comes in quite handy as a nurse.

Once you get to the floor you will run into these issues. Whether you view them as a blessing or curse is wholly up to you. I looked at them for the gifts they bring more than anything else.

As an older nurse: You look more mature so people think you have been a nurse forever. As such, they expect that you will know how to do procedures you have never done. They will expect you know how to handle things you may feel shaky with and they will expect that you move with the quickness of an experienced nurse. Getting help from a peer, stutter stepping in a task and hesitation makes your patient and their family doubt you and doubt you hard.

You are at the bottom of the totem pole again. Remember that ladder that you spent so much time climbing in your old job? The one you swore you would never climb again? Well, here it is and you need to start climbing because you are on the bottom again. You have to take the crappy shifts, you are the outsider, you are the one that needs to work you ass off; again.

Suck it up + work hard. Period.

Your ego can take a large beating here if you let it. The first time someone tells you what to do, or there is some new rule you have to follow that doesn't make any sense to you it will be tough especially if you spent any time in your 'other' career being the boss. You are going to want to 'right fight' it; resist that urge and things will run more smoothly for you.

You see redundancy quicker. As someone with experience, it is easy to see inefficiency in the processes that are happening on the floor you go to work on. Please do not assume that they want to hear your feedback on how to improve things and make them better. Do not think it is a good idea to show them their inefficiency or deficits straight up just because you can see them so clearly. No one likes to be told their stuff sucks, you know? They may ask you to tell them and they may even have a little sign up at the door that asks for suggestions.

Be careful with the way you ride in and try to save the day here. You are going to work here for a while and you want them to like you. Be gentle and creative in the way you share your thoughts. It might even help to give them info via one of the charge nurses and let that wonderful idea be theirs instead of yours. You do not really care how it gets done or who gets credit for it, you just want it changed

The 12 hour shifts are a little bit harder. Wear support socks. Buy some kick ass shoes. Drink plenty of water and do not hold your bladder. If you need to pee then do it. (**Note to Self**: Enforce this rule-pee when needed!) Bring your lunch and make it something healthy. Your patients will not even guess that you are a new nurse. So unless you tell them they will trust you a lot more quickly than your 25 year old counterpart.

Use that power wisely. While you are at it, use your life experience to help those kiddos out. Show them how to juggle tasks, help them learn to laugh at things and let go of what is not important. Over all, being a 2nd career nurse helped me transition with a bit of ease that only life experience brings. I don't sweat the small stuff.

When you are overwhelmed try this; stop. breathe, smile. It is better than Xanax to calm your nerves

Things are never as bad as you think they are

MANAGEMENT MISCHIEF

Just a small word about this only because I know it will come up at some point as you get to know things on your unit.

Smiley General may help people heal and all just don't forget that this is a corporation. Even the non-profit groups want to make or at the least not lose money.

Management and their politics are everywhere.

I spent a lot of time in the corporate world before I started to study nursing. I climbed the hierarchy until I was at the top of the ladder. It was tough for me to be okay with all the decision-making that happened under the guise of being 'for the people' that actually had very little to do 'with' the people.

At first, I really believed that the work I did made a difference for folks. Somewhere over the years that belief took a backseat to feeling like a total sleaze. I mean, I no longer felt like I was doing work that mattered to anything but the boss's pocket. It was hard to reconcile telling customers that they mattered when I knew that the reality was that the financial bottom-line was the most important item discussed in the director's meeting we held each week. At some point I suppose, everything is about the money.

For me, spinning lies so they appeared truth made me physically ill., so I hung up the business hat and went back to school to become a nurse.

While I was fulfilling a life-long dream, I had painted such a gorgeous picture of what nursing was like in my head that I did not even stop and think there would be politics in this world, too.

All I could see was the focus on the patient and the feeling that this was actually work that mattered. I never factored in corporate anything.

It was my first week of school, I was asked by a professor to explain why I had left the high-pay and high-power corporate world. There were, she explained, many nurses choosing to leave the bedside in favor of roles similar to the one I had abandoned.
That was easy; I had left the corporate world because I did not want to 'be in the middle of politics' anymore.

Her reaction was more negative than I expected.

She could not see the same altruism within nursing as I could not see any good in corporate design. She was quick to adjust the wind in my sails.

Hospitals are huge businesses filled with politics on many, many levels. Even those that 'say' they are not for profit, unfortunately, are still watching profit. Adding a layer of always changing regulation in place to protect patient's, the fact that you deal with life and death each day and the many strong personalities jockeying for position in the hospital left me in larger politically charged environment that what I had just left..

Hmmm, as you can imagine this was not good news to me at all; still I am not naïve about business.

I knew that there was always politics and always ego and always bottom-line. I resolved right then and there to never allow that to be a driving force in the work that I did as a nurse, the way it had in the corporate world.

Fast-forward to the first thirty days of employment at Smiley

General. Whew, there was a lot of corporate rhetoric. It is the same everywhere. The mission statement and mottos designed to unite us in a common goal were presented over and over again. Most people could get on board with them because they made common sense. It was more or less the Golden Rule stated in hundreds of different ways.

Some of my experienced peers in orientation were offended by the time it took for them to explain things to us that any 10 yr old could figure out. Easy to see that they were just covering their butt by saying they 'had informed us', still I hated the time suck.

I was offended a little later than my new peers by the amount fear used to coerce me into completing education packets or change the way I gave care. It made me upset to see emails asking us to follow some new evidence in our practice and then see a large portion of staff not follow the rule and also see nothing done about it.

It made me ask the question in my head almost daily 'is {fillintheblankwiththenewrule} important or not?'

If it is then enforce the rule if not then do not make the rule....

Then there is the whole continuing education, thing.

You know, medicine is constantly advancing and as it does the way we practice changes. This is one of the things I loved the most when I went into nursing-I was assured I would not ever be bored.

So, there are a lot of different kinds of education. You get some from within Smiley General and some from higher learning institutes. You will always have this or that module to complete regarding HIPAA or Ethics and you will always be asked to keep getting the next highest level of education; this I totally get. It is the presentation that is rough to handle.

See, if you ask most nurses they are going to tell you that education is uber important to them. They want to learn things relevant to their practice, though.

They will tell you that they recognize the value of evidence-based practice and they want to use that evidence to provide the best care possible for their patient. Most of us even want to pursue education on the outside.

If you force an ADN nurse into getting her BSN by insinuation that she is not good enough to care for patients while that ADN nurse is busting hump and working circles around more educated peeps, well, you are going to decrease morale; especially when that ADN nurse has been nursing for 15 plus years.

You would think the mucky-mucks could see how demoralizing it is; it happens though.

All of this chat to say simply, there will be at least one point in the first few months of your new nursing gig when you stop and wonder what kind of corporate cog you have become.

You will wonder if anyone else can see cross purposes in the emails between bosses. There will be a time or two when you have to ask in order to clarify which new 'rule' takes precedence when they contradict one another. The mandatory education modules you are asked to complete will not always teach you anything new.

The irony of all the emails and items that tell you patient care is our focus while creating more steps that are not about patient care will not be hard to spot at your level. The uppers don't always see how adding spreadsheets to report patient care add to your time away from patient care.

Regardless, make an effort to step away from the frustration and focus on what you came to do; care for patients.

Do what you need to do in order to rise above the politics of the system while working within the system.

I knew a battle on this front would not serve me and still I had to work hard to let it go. I am supposing that was because I had been in management and I could see how detrimental it was to our objective. I loved this place and the patients and my new peers so I wanted everything to be right and 'non-corporate' dontchaknow.

It was worth the time it took to let it go though.

Here are a few things that might help you in this effort.

Tips for Maneuvering around Management

- o Ignore politics. You have a nursing practice to craft and patients to see.
- o Don't take anything personally. This will keep the chip off your shoulder.
- o Don't spend energy complaining about rules or regulations. It will not change anything.
- o Remember that you are all after what is best for patients.
- o If you have a valid issue then do something with it in a valid way; take it to a manager for review.
- o If you have a unit counsel or other nurse-led governance body then become a part of that group.

- You have to put the role of management in the right perspective in order to remain unaffected by the politics and you have to remember that you are going to get what you expect to get from every situation.
- Examine your own feelings before you say a word.
- Make an effort to compliment people on the good you seeing them do. You can't focus on negative if you are focused on being awesome!

All-in-all I would say that management means well with all the rules they make + that they care about patients as much as we do; they just come at it from a different angle is all. The governing bodies truly act to keep patients safe. They just don't focus on the practicality of their rules the way we do.

This is one of those areas that you should not spend time focused on; it just wastes your time.

Unless you plan to jump into it and change it from the inside out. If that is your fight to fight then I say 'go get 'em tiger!'

Focus Point: You have to put yourself on the same team as management even if you do not agree with them. You are all after what is best for the patient, after all.

Action Step: Find one thing that you like about the way things are run on your floor and focus on this when something crazy comes down the pike.

Mantra Mojo: *I am centered on patient care. My ego is not attached to how things are done for the patient only that the best care is taken of that patient.*

THE POWER OF DISENGAGEMENT

There is going to be some stress these first months.

I am pretty sure you expected it.

So let me ask you, what things do you do to de-stress yourself?

Do you do them regularly to keep stress at bay or do you do them only after you're overflowing with emotion + crankiness? Do you have to get to that place before you realize you are internalizing stress?

What type of personality do you have, Nurse Awesome? Do you wear your heart on your sleeve? Do you cry or yell often? Do you get your feelings hurt easily or do you let things roll right off you like water off a duck's back?

I want you to be honest with yourself about these answers.

This is probably the most important chapter in this book.

Cause if you are going to be at this stuff long-term it is critical for you to figure out how to disengage from your nursing practice and your patient population. Unplugging, relaxing, de-stressing, whatever you call it. You gotta have a way to tune into your own vibe and see what you need to do to remain healthy and balanced.

The ability to do this is as important as any other thing you can learn in your first year as a nurse.

I didn't pay much attention here and it jumped up to bite me, hard.

The way I view it now is like this:

Learning how to take great care of me is the ONLY way that I am going to be able to take great care of the WORLD.

Reread that last sentence.
To date, I have been super-great at taking care of the world; me not quite as much.

Nursing is an emotionally charged profession that is also physically, mentally and spiritually demanding.

Sure, there were situations in school that were tough to handle. The volume of information that comes at you in a typical day in nursing school can leave you feeling like an avalanche has just buried you, right? Drug information, procedure instructions, skills testing, body systems and disease process, communication techniques; the list could go on for days. Not to mention the family stress of having to lock yourself away to study.

No small wonder that we leave school feeling so damn 'full'.

Nursing 'for real' leaves you with a different feeling from school altogether. It is still quite 'full'.

I didn't find myself in many spots during school that a good belly laugh or time with friends wouldn't erase. I knew in school that eventually I would be done with it and the stress that came with it would therefore, also be gone.

I attacked school with this hyper-focus. I got told a lot the first semester that I needed to 'lighten up'. I wanted to leave school with a 4.0 GPA but more importantly than that I wanted to leave as a nurse that would be fully prepared for any patient situation that I may face in those first months after school.

Funny enough, I did not succeed at either the 4.0 or the being prepared to handle every patient situation. Ha!

I put a lot of pressure on myself to be perfect because I took the job of maintaining life seriously and I was super-intense in my pursuit of perfection.
While I would be done with school eventually, I would never be done with my career. So, I took that intensity into my first job.

Hello, Critical Care is an area that you need to take seriously!

I was working on the floor and in a residency program that required class time 2 days a week. In between, I was studying the new contraptions I was working with and busy learning the new drugs that ICU brings and preparing for the AACN certification.

I was leaving work tired both physically and mentally. Some days totally overwhelmed spiritually. There was something else too. Despite all the study I was doing I walked into work every day feeling certain I would kill someone. I waited for it. In fact, I just 'knew' that my lack of perfection was going to end a human life.

I can throw on a confident swagger when needed so I did a great job hiding it however; underneath there was a constant feeling that I was going to lose my shit at any moment.

I was on the verge of tears by shift end on most days for the first month. I felt like I was walking around with a hundred pound weight on my chest all the time. I was questioning myself about every little thing I did and all of it was stressing me out. It took me the entire 3 days off to recover then I was right back in the mire again. I was not happy but I did not really know why I was unhappy.

I felt kinda like a brat because I had finished school and gotten the job I dreamed of having so really, why on EARTH was I feeling so low? What the hell was wrong with me!

I spent some time batting it around my brain for a few days and finally decided to ask for some help. I mentioned the feelings of inadequacy I was feeling to my preceptor and asked how to prevent it. Her reply was simple...'sorry toots, you can't.' She went on to tell me:

> 'if you walk around here all the time hesitating because you are afraid you will kill someone or obsessing over trying to be perfect in every little thing you do then you are going to make yourself insane really fast. You need to just accept something right now. People die here. You are not working at Wal-Mart. You are in hospital and in an ICU, they were sick as shit when they got here, you did not make them that way and they might die, again something that is not in your hands. You can only do the best you can do and you must, must, must let that be enough'

Word....

It took me a few days to digest that statement. I had a hard time reconciling it between my head and my heart. There were a lot of really tragic patients those few months. We cared for many young people with sudden and horrific outcomes. I got the medical examiner's phone number stuck in my memory that first month and spent lots of time on the county medical examiner website reviewing cause of death and looking at obituary columns.

I did post-mortem care on people my kids age and it was damn tough for my right-brained, wide-opened heart to process. (**Note to Self**: you can cry if you need)

It took me awhile to reframe what my preceptor was saying to me.

However you adapt, please understand that bad shit will happen despite your best intentions. You can be stressed about it and it will happen. You can do the best you can and it will happen. You can let go of it and it will happen. Bad things will happen. Let's lay that aside and focus on what we can change, shall we?

The focus point is simply this: you have to get rid of what stresses you rather than letting it linger in your body. There is not any way that you can operate in the environment of nursing for long without beginning to wear some of your patients suffering yourself. Your heart is broken for them. Your mind spins from the possible implications that a similar event could have in your own life. You wonder 'what-if' this had been you, your mom, dad, child etc.
You start to read obituaries. You start to call and check on patients on your days off. While these are understandably human choices; in excess these are not healthy behaviors.

I repeat: It is not healthy to check the obituaries daily for past patients. (**Note to Self**: The Medical Examiner website is also not relaxing-stop looking at it.)

Each shift has the potential to leave you feeling fulfilled and as if you actually 'did' matter that day.

Each shift also has the potential to leave you feeling like nothing you did made any difference at all.

I guess I was 3 months into my career in the ICU when I stopped trying to figure out why the school I went to focused so little on helping me prepare for how emotionally drained I would feel at the end of the day. To me, that was just as important as the other skill we were so rigorously tested on in skills lab.

I could recall conversations about how to handle the patients feelings, lots of therapeutic communication techniques were learned, but I don't seem to recall anyone telling me how to deal with my own feelings.

There was instruction about every topic imaginable but nothing that told me how to keep my mind and my heart from playing dodge ball with one another every day.

I had gathered lots of tricks to help my patients cope but was sorely lacking in tricks to help myself.
There is a huge assumption that you already 'know' how to keep your emotions in check and that you have the emotional intelligence to sort out your feelings 'post event' and carry on.

Smiley General assumes it through your orientation period.

You may be wondering why the assumptions, huh?

Here's the thing, regardless of our GPA, the program we came from or our previous life experience the system you are about to enter, aka Smiley General Hospital, thinks we are awesome hires, right? Sure! That is why they picked us to join them.

So while that is great and all, part of our awesomeness is that we already know how to thrive in the crazy transition from student to registered nurse. At least that is what

Smiley General believes.

It innocently forgets to factor in how many things that only experience can teach us. It just doesn't consider it might need to help us work through the intense level of both relief + stress that come with the knowledge that we are finally working under our own license. ***Note to Self***: don't forget to protect your license

It believes that passing our NCLEX means we can adapt quickly + that we can handle all the hard bits of humanness we're about to encounter on our path.

It's an easy assumption to make, after all. Smiley General knows that we come with a great education. It knows we have tons of enthusiasm + love for this profession and that we take patient care personally.

I've watched many nurses crumble under the weight of the emotional stuff that gets stuffed because they either lack the tools to process it or lack the self-care skills that recognize it as something that they need to let go. I've watched them lose their passion for patient care before they even fully understand the power of their presence.

All of which could have been avoided had they known how to check in with their soul to see if they were full or not and had planned a strategy to correct it once they identified it.

So, maybe you can't recognize the feeling of full just yet.

What you CAN do is to realize that your cup 'will runneth over' and that you will need some tools to help you empty it.

The first meltdown you have should leave you thinking, 'Ah heck, I let my cup get to full!'

You have to find a way to disengage from the suffering and plug back into what fuels you as a human being before you can be a kick ass nurse.

Everyone is different so the fuel you pick may look nothing like mine. The tools you use may look nothing like mine. Just know that whatever you pick you need something you can practice <u>daily</u> that gets rid of that days stress as well as a pouch full of other tools to practice <u>weekly</u> that help you plug back into your soul again.

Using the tools you determine will work for you and keeping up with practicing them will keep you centered and peaceful and healthy as a new nurse. Mostly.

Think of it as Boy Scout training for nurses. You gotta be prepared!

So, funny thing, I have been teaching people the importance of emptying their internal cup + disengaging from stress since I was about 25; I was more than shocked when I found myself in need of some disengagement.

I really never thought I would be 'the one' to take things home with me.

My husband was the first to notice. 'You don't seem like yourself' he said casually one day. He also commented on the fact that we had not been on a ride in while. He knows this is one of my favorite ways to dump stress. His observations only annoyed me.

My son, the second to notice, 'Mom, where is that positive outlook of yours run off to? You seem really moody lately'. It was true that my usual funny-sarcastic side had lost its fun. Truth was I felt like a rubber-band that was stretched super-tight all day. It just took one little touch to make me jump all over the place. I loved my job but I hated going each day because I hated that I could not control the outcome for my patients.

Among other things.

I finally got to feeling so overwhelmed that I was forced to take a closer look at my issues. It was hard to admit I had any issues at all given that I was super-nursing student, you know?

When I got still about it and quit saying I 'was fine' I could see pretty clearly what was happening. (N*ote to Self*: saying the word fine a lot means you better get some help!)

I was in serious need of disengagement. My cup was full and when I could not hold anymore stress, sadness, delays, cranky patients, cranky families I would begin to feel horrible.

I really did not think that was even something was possible for me because already took active steps weekly to unplug from life and rid myself of stress. Disengage to me meant 'stop caring' which was not really true at all.

Did you know that the word nurse is derived from the phrase 'to nourish'? I didn't although I did know that most nurses are nurturers. Nurturing means I care. I could not think about a point in time when I could 'stop' caring for my patients so it was logical to conclude that I would always be stuck miserable and worrying about them.

When you started nursing school you may not have considered caring about your patient population and their families to be a problem. In fact, it was most likely a motivator for you to start nursing school in the first place.

Let's see if any of these sound familiar to you.

> I want a profession where I feel like my efforts matter

> I want to make a difference in peoples' lives.

> I wanted to change the world.

> I have always been the caretaker of people so I figured I may as well be paid for doing it, right?'

> I just love people so it was a natural choice.

Even though nursing is a noble calling it exposes you to the highs and lows of human existence every single shift. You don't have to work in ICU to feel it.

At this point, I started cutting my school some slack for neglecting to teach me how to cope. There is not really any way to prepare you for the real world while you are in school because you cannot know the stress of the space fully until you get into the space fully.

So now that you know it is going to happen, what are your going to do to help yourself stay centered?

What can you do to help yourself disengage at the end of each shift?

How will you keep from checking the obituary column on your day off? Any ideas?

You know, how are you going to unplug, unwind, give up the thought you can control any of it and actually leave work at work?

Think about it for a while. I surely did.

Once I got over my own ego saying that I was 'above' getting sucked into the emotional aspect of my job it was easy to find some things that helped me. Many of my 'tools' have evolved into very grounding routines for me. Sort of the way that a toddler needs a set routine for bedtime to get to sleep well; I needed these disengagement rituals to be the happiest me.

Don't freak out. People have been using rituals for centuries to bring order to their world. Religions of all sorts are packed with ritual. Even school systems and corporations carry on their affairs in a ritual-like manner.

I did a fair amount of ceremony in school. I lit candles and prayed before tests, I ate the same breakfast every day before clinical. I sat in the same study room + chair in the library; I used the same color pens. I am sure you did these things too. So just turn the page on those rituals of school and let them morph into new rituals that you can count on to boost your morale and disconnect your emotions from your patients at the end of shift. Let go of any aversion you feel towards the word ritual. Insert the word ceremony, mantra, meditation, self-care, practice; whatever you need to actually do it.

The first ritual I developed after noticing how full I was getting on each shift centered on a colorful beaded bracelet that I used to wear when I was afraid. No one but me knew that I was shoring myself up from fear when I wore it (although I guess they will now). Didn't matter though, because I knew, right? It was cheap enough that I could wear it at work and it could get wet or cootied up or ruined or whatever and so I started wearing it every night during my shift. I was afraid a lot!

Here are all the 'rituals' I have developed over the last year of nursing. I call them tools and as silly and unrelated to nursing as some of them seem, they really help. Keep in mind a ritual can be anything that you do with intention that carries a meaning behind it. No need for fancy. The meanings I share underneath each action are solely mine so feel free to adapt them to your needs.

You don't have to wait until your shift ends to disengage from the stress you are feeling

In fact, it is preferable that you do not wait until then but do this as the day unfolds.

I can be seen stretching frequently at 0200. I am known to dance while pulling meds or boogie my way with the IV pole to the storage closet.

I am not crazy. It is me letting go of stress intentionally as much as taking care of my back.

What do you do now to relieve stress?

List those things here:

Tools I Use to Prepare for shift

aka switch from plain old-Melissa into Nurse Awesome

1. I don't think about work until I get to work. There is nothing I can do about it anyway
2. I keep my badge in the car and I don't strap on those brilliant RN initials on until I get to work. There is usually some exclamation that goes with this act, 'Let's rock this B*&%$!' is a favorite.
3. Right after that exclamation comes a short prayer-A symbol that now I am stepping into the role of nurse. 'let me be a beneficial presence' is all I ask
4. Put on my watch and a bracelet that I have deemed my 'magic' bracelet. It connects me in an instant to the greatest minds of all time which I may need thru my shift-my peers have heard me more than once as I touch my bracelet mutter, 'no sweat I just need to channel my inner Einstein or my Inner Flo'
5. I fill my pockets with my 'stuff'(stethoscope, hemostats and what not) until I get to the break room right before shift. In doing this I am silently telling the Universe that I have 'everything I need' to have an ass-kicking shift. After all, these are the tools of my superpower and batman never wears his utility belt when he is Bruce Wayne.

Tools I use to Disengage from the Energy of My Shift-aka morph back into plain old-Melissa

I empty my pockets at the nurses' station before I leave. Don't need these powerful tools when I a tools when I am not being a nurse. This tells my brain, okay, it is time to stop being Nurse Awesome, honey.

1. I go pee before I leave the floor. I make a point of always going pee when I need to (unless my patient is crashing) this is a silent affirmation that I matter. Doing it right before I leave is just a symbol that I am now in taking care of me mode-not taking care of patients' mode.
2. I hum out loud and smile on my way to my car. A symbol that 'all is well' in my world.
3. I say thank you over and over as I hum Gratitude for being allowed to be a beneficial presence is important.
4. I remove my name badge once I get into the car It goes in the same place so I can reclaim my power quickly
5. I remove my superpower bracelet before I turn on the car: The last symbol for me before I go home. It says simply ' Now I am simply Melissa not Super Nurse who just took care of dying people'

Other Tools I use to keep my balance during my shift

I do these things often; you can try some of these or find your own. I love to laugh and am fairly silly + sarcastic so that is the reason these are playful in nature. Whatever works for you. I just worked with one awesome nurse that uses her hand washing as a chance to wash the entire funk away. As she counts her own blessings she regains her center. I am finding that they not only help me stay empty but they help me be a better human. That ultimately helps me be a better nurse.

Etch-A-Sketch-Yes, I carry a tiny one with me and I use it when I am stressed to draw on, then when I shake it up and down I pretend I am releasing all the negative thoughts I am having about that particular shift or situation. I used it a LOT when I was a brand new nurse. Not so much anymore but then, yes, I needed frequent release of stress to keep me from losing my shit.

Soul Train Dance Party-Sometimes the only way to wash the funk away is to get funky! Pick your favorite groove tune and hum it while you work. Shake your booty at the Pyxis, Bust a move in the supply room. Any way that you can to readjust the haze that has built up around your awesome. I have been busted actually strutting to a room on more than one occasion. Extra points if you pick a song everyone remembers and get the whole unit singing along!

Magic Door Memory Eraser-We walk through these big glass doors into our patients' rooms. I play this game with myself, especially when families or patients are extremely tough. I imagine as I pass through the door that a large blast of air sweeps away all the stuff these tough people just hurled at me. Sort of like the wind blaster at the automatic carwash. Don't laugh; it works to keep a ton of negative emotions and sarcastic comments from becoming reality out in the open.

Magic Wand-As in I carry one in my nursing bag? You really never know when you need some magic,right? Truly this reminds me to laugh, it reminds me of my own power, and it reminds me that when I am plugged into my Source (aka God) there is magic that never leaves me.

Prayer or Meditation-I ask for help with all my tasks and I release my patients at shift end. At some point, usually once I have met my patient, I ask every angel around me to help me be a beneficial presence and not cause harm. I actually say the mantras I suggest to you through this book. Try it.

Setting intention for each shift-I think good thoughts and know that each thing I need will show up as I need it. Don't underestimate the power in this simple act. I actually think setting intention for a great shift is one of the most powerful things I can do.

Asking for guidance when I am in the patients room- As a newbie I was not always sure of my role, so I asked for help from all the unseen forces around me(yes I believe in angels) so I would know what part of my nursing skills will be most beneficial to them in each moment them.
There are others I use in a pinch however; these things happen at frequent intervals depending on how I feel.

You really have to be in touch with your own feelings in order to determine if your energy is getting wonky. If you are not sure how to tell just start by noticing how you feel.

Are you happy or sad going into work?

Do you feel stressed with no cause you can pinpoint?

Do you feel uplifted by the work that you do in the world?

Are you still as eager to nurse as you were in school?

Ask a friend or your spouse to help you gauge where your

energy is during this transition from school.

A lot of stress vanishes once you hang up your student badge. You do get some different stress in its place but that stress does not have to run your life. It does not have to change you.

Smiley General is going to assume you know how to handle your emotions without having a breakdown however; I am asking you not to make the same assumptions with your mental health. If you feel crappy, stop long enough to share that with someone, please. Then investigate all this emotional stuff even if you are not particularly bent toward emotion. We all get full, even those who have nerves of steel need emotional release.

Take some time to develop a few tools, habits, and rituals; whatever you want to call them. Use them for the purpose of disengaging from the energy of your patient and their families. If you use them often you will find the suffering you watch does not attach itself to you and weight you down and that you are able to leave your worry in the shift instead of taking it home with you.

Take your own emotional pulse every day to see when you need to make adjustments to the routine or take some time off. There is a lot you cannot control in your shift but this emotional health thing is something that you are totally controlling. Focus on what you can do to give yourself more power mentally and emotionally instead of all the things going wrong. **Note to Self:** What shows up for you in your shift will follow your thoughts so pay attention to them.

Nurses are known for caring. That is all well and good, you just have to figure out how to take care of your own needs while busy meeting the needs of your patients each shift. If you find yourself feeling 'off' and just cannot put a finger on where that is coming from, failing to disengage you from your patient might just be the culprit.

Focus Point: It is hard to watch other people suffer on the daily and not carry some of that home with you. Our job description forgets to mention that we will be carrying an enormous amount of stress. Finding a way to unload that stress and taking great care of you is the only way that you can take great care of the world.

Action Step: Figure out how to disengage your energy, your heart, your soul from the lives you are caring for each shift. There are 100's of ways to do it. Just pick something and do it consistently.

Mantra Mojo: Allow me to be a beneficial presence in all that I do.

CRAFTING YOUR INDIVIDUAL PRACTICE

We spent a lot of time in school being homogenized into evidence-based practice robots so this next piece of conversation is going to seem a bit odd at first. Stay with me though, I think it will fit like a glove once we get done chatting.

This chapter is about making your new nursing practice as far from homogenized as possible. It is about expressing yourself fully through your actions with your patients while at the same time keeping those evidenced-based rules and board regulations that we all must follow.

Individual practice + evidence-based practice are not mutually exclusive. Nothing in the awesome nurse rulebook says you must give up self-expression in order to be an awesome nurse.

In truth it is the other way around, infusing your whole self in your nursing career is just as essential as that stethoscope around your neck.

Crafting your practice is not an activity that happens on the surface. You have to go deeper than what school or society at large encourages, by that I mean that you have to be willing to look at what motivates you to do what you do; you need to know the 'real why' behind *why* you nurse. That answer may not be on the surface. It may take some work to get to the place where you truly feel like your nursing practice is a true reflection of you.

It is not impossible at all and not particularly hard to achieve. It just requires you pay attention and invest time in yourself for a change.

Note to Self: no stress here-there is plenty of time to get comfy with the day-to-day operations before you venture to this place.

At this point in the chapter you might be wondering what on earth 'infusing you' in your practice has to do with anything.
To be painfully honest, it has everything to do with it.

I have worked with more than a couple nurses that have been nurses for a long time. I have mad respect for all the nursing knowledge they have crammed in their head that effortlessly appears at the exact moment it is needed. What they also had, and what they asked for help with from me, was a pervasive pissiness towards patients, management, and just about anything related to the profession they once loved.

Most of them have a king-sized chip on their shoulder and walk around waiting for it to be knocked off. Look around your floor when you get there. They are the nurses that do not help anyone else, that gripe about every task on their list, that constantly fall behind and that leave you feeling like you need a bath after listening to all the negative that comes from them.

So the common theme among them is two-fold.

Failing to refill their cup, giving too much of themselves to the profession and their patients so nothing is left for themselves is a huge factor.

The other half of it has invariably been that they do not view their practice as an expression of themselves. They are not personally invested anymore therefore it is not important to them any longer. They do not look at nursing as a way to share their best parts with the world. It is only a revenue stream not a passion the way it was in the beginning.

So you have a choice, you can believe it now or wait till you prove it to yourself some years down the road, your longevity in this career, if not sanity, depends on your willingness to view your practice as a living 'thing' rather than just a job you do each day.

This will make sure that YOU are represented as much as Smiley General in YOUR practice and opens the way for some sacred connections to form between you and your patient. That connection is the fuel that you need to keep going when everything else leaves you empty.
Crafting your practice is about actively nourishing your nursing career + your spirit with the same passion you give to patient care.

It is letting your spirit free fall into your practice with no piece left aside so that your patients get the best parts of you every day. That is where your medicine lives; in the best parts of you.

While it is hard to imagine as you run around trying to stay afloat in this transition to your new job, all the pieces of you are vital to your patients' recovery, and to your own personal health.

Crafting you practice is about raising the bar for yourself and then expecting other nurses to meet you there, that takes some crazy devotion on your part. Once you find what is important to you in your practice you have to work at making it non-negotiable. As in, you MUST focus on these things in your practice each shift. No matter how much shit is hitting the fan, this center will hold.

The only way that you can sustain the kind of devotion I am

talking about here is to abso-total-lutely love, love, LOVE the heck outta what you are doing.

Do you love the type of nursing you are doing?

As a new nurse it may be tough to tell at first. A few months in and you will know if you have found your nursing home. Until then, never mind that you are a new nurse, your practice is still a living thing and needs to be infused with the essence of you!

Let's put our toes in the surf and see how the water feels.

Check in with your gut right now, superstar.
What did you feel as I suggested you infuse your practice with your own spirit and personality?

What kind of thoughts went through your head?

Did it open you up or shut you down?

Did you think, 'that sounds lovely'

Or

Did you think, 'this chick is a nut job'

The answer only matters to you. Come back to those questions as you gain some experience and see how your feelings change. Use that as a gauge to know when you are ready to begin infusing your practice with the wonderment of you.

I spent 20 years dreaming of the day I would finally get to practice nursing for a living so you can damn sure bet I had a detailed vision of what it would be like in real-life. I've told you already about the visions of Florence Nightingale dancing in my head. I was not exaggerating.

In addition to those visions, I just knew that as a nurse I would leave at the end of each day with a sense of pride + fulfillment that no other job could give me. I thought it would be easy to throw my heart into my job since I did that with many other areas of my life.

I believed that my patients would feel valued and that they would appreciate the thoughtful care I gave them + my hearts ability to love. I just never realized how much work it would take to do it or how little support I would find while claiming a practice that was uniquely my own..

School was not the place for revealing your heart. It was much, much harder than it needed to be for many reasons we cannot get into here, let's just say it was hard to see the value of my heart there. Not much made me feel appreciated in my brief clinical days; let alone was there any room for my best traits to engage. Every time I tried to do that I was pretty quickly squashed like a bug.
As I moved into the real-world and began to feel a bit more balance + a little less 'squashable' I could see the potential for my daydream to become real.

Even before my NCLEX was done my spirit was getting excited to come out and play in this new role, you know, to create the career I had envisioned.

I was surprised to find that individuality was talked about but not so much encouraged within in the walls of Smiley General. My peer groups had the same stories from their employers so my perspective was not the exception.

I started my practice with excitement oozing out my pores. I quickly noticed many of those long-term nurses I adored did not love their job at all. They did not feel blessed by their ability to help other humans and worse yet, did not see the value in the contribution they made each day. There was little in their practice that they could truly call a reflection of their soul.

This blew my mind! How could someone saving and changing lives not see their contribution? How could someone with the special and unique skill set it takes to be a nurse long-term feel any way other than blessed? I was in awe of them, why were they not in awe of themselves?

Even some of my own school peer group were questioning whether or not they mattered from a pretty quick place after starting work. It broke my heart into a million little pieces to hear a brand new nurse already making plans to leave the bedside.

I'm not sure how it got that way, a combination of customer service nursing and corporate fluff I suspect. These effectively reduce the nurse to being a medicine concierge at the Hilton where customer service and high nurse to patient ratios trump patient safety or nurse instinct. It could be the weight of ridiculous rules that are never enforced or extra steps for the nurse for the sake of reporting, rather than patient care, that cause a nurses spirit to crumble. Might even be providing radical + invasive (read painful) care to patients that are going to die despite your efforts; essentially rendering your butt-busting pointless.

There is no need to get into any of that here, corporations do what works for them; just like people do and overall my employer was a good one that was doing what worked for them. Focusing on the only thing you can control, yourself, is better than attempting to change the system at this point.

Having control over you is wholly empowering.

The bottom line is that healthcare is filled with nurses that hate their job and this translates to patient care. Nursing is filled with well-meaning researchers who spend gobs of time developing evidence-based studies that tell us how to best nourish our patients but fail to tell us how to nourish ourselves in the middle of all we do to nourish the patient. It is a slippery slope.

Nourishing yourself is essential and something totally up to you, starshine. In order to fully nourish yourself you have to learn to disengage from patients(we've done that part)and you have to learn what is important to you. Once you learn it and you start to nurse consciously and consistently from that place no amount of craziness or corporate 'stuff' can take the joy away from your job.

A few more reasons to craft your own practice:
- Being inauthentic makes you crabby + crabby sucks!
- Negativity eventually creates disease or 'dis-ease'
- Stressful environments do not encourage self-care and a hungry nurse that needs to pee is a nurse that is distracted and cranky + will make mistakes in patient care
- Nurses that bring their whole heart to their practice are happier and happier nurses do not job hop creating better healing space for patients
- Eventually all of us end up in the system. Do you want yourself and your loved ones taken care of by a nurse that that has no passion left for nursing?

It sucks to leap into your new career filled with love of people and a huge passion for the science of nursing only to feel drained of that passion shortly thereafter so what can we do to change it?

It has to start with a shift in our individual mindset

which will influence the collective mindset. In English, huh?

We have to focus on our own heart in our own practice.

We have to make some lists of things we 'must-do' as a nurse and a human and that we 'must-have' from an employer and then we have to set about getting those lists fulfilled.

Yes, I am serious. You need to start by knowing what traits feel essential to you, what things you want to leave behind with your patient.

Even at this stage in your young career you have every right to work someplace that resonates with the overall theme of what you want to express, too!

I know that seems like an odd thing to say since we are led to believe we just have to 'take what we get' and shut our mouth about the rest. If you go to work somewhere that does not resonate with your own personal vibe, regardless of the reason, you should make plans to leave that place soon. Take it from an old lady-it is not worth the love you lose to stay.

I know you are wondering how in the world you are supposed to 'craft your practice'. Ah, let's you and I open some dialogue about that, shall we?

This is a good place to start.

Truly embrace that this is YOUR practice to do with what makes your heart sing. This is easy for some people and super-tough for others. Don't judge yourself about it.

Every day for a month, just before you go into shift, I want you to say out loud to yourself.

'This is MY nursing practice and I get to express the best parts of me here.'

Let it be easy, there is not a right or wrong way to go about this; it is just gentle exploration is all.

Now then, notice where your thoughts are about your practice. Do you see it as an extension of you? What did you feel as you said those few words to claim your space? Did it feel uneasy?

It might feel odd and that is okay. The thought that you don't have to homogenize yourself and be like everyone else is strange I know.

Crafting your practice can start in earnest as soon as you pass that NCLEX exam. Your license confirms that you are capable of keeping a patient safe and alive while in your care.

So that is not an issue. We are talking about how you stay connected to this career you chose for the long-haul.

For example, one of the things at the top of my own list is that I express kindness in my practice. I do not always get it right. Some of the more colorful folks I care for sure make me work at it. One thing I am certain of is that regardless of the external stimuli they provide it is up to me to flip it, twist it, or otherwise morph it so that what comes out of me regardless of their input is kind.
I am willing to make that effort if I need to, I am willing to do the work, hold my tongue, and smile when I want to scream.

I do those things because kindness matters to me and as such I view it as an essential part of my own nursing practice. If I remove kindness than I remove a piece of me from the equation and doing that, over the long haul, will make me cranky, resentful, bitter and all kinds of mean. Much more so than letting go of the need to correct a crazy patient.

See what I mean? On the surface, in that moment, it seems like venting to a co-worker or crabbing about that patient in some way will be the best choice. It is a temporary solution, it is ego driven. It will make me feel vindicated for a half a minute is all. If I take the whole minute and look deeper I see it is not good for me to put that kind of stuff out into the world again, because kindness matters to me. (***Note to Self***: practice not perfect)

It doesn't matter what type of nursing I do, I view it as an expression of my heart, soul and mind and I've no doubt that the way I choose to express myself is something in my complete control.

Look, the healthcare system we occupy likes homogenous nurses because sameness allows easy measure. It is predictable and easier to capture on a survey score.

Here is the rub...You were born as an individual expression of divinity so there is not any way possible you can show up in the world like everyone else-at least not for the long term. There are countless reasons people leave their personality + heart out of things at Smiley General. Most of it boils down to either not realizing it was 'okay' to be themselves or feeling scared to death the parts they show will be squashed.

Either way it is crazy important to learn not to hide your heart and the beliefs you value from your practice. Practice allowing rather than excluding pieces of your heart and soul while you practice.

Another simple example: my patients are not always conscious however; every single shift I make sure at least once that I tell them how much their presence on earth matters. I also always thank my patients for allowing me to care for them, tell them they were a blessing and wish them well; even if this is a whisper in their ear as I leave shift.

I don't do this because it's part of our unit protocol, although I am sure some new rule about it will come soon, I do it because it is important to me that people know they matter and that they know I appreciated their presence in our sacred space.

So you spent some time before shift claiming that this was YOUR practice and you did that for 30 days. Awesome!

Now take some time to set the intent before your shift that you are going to be fully present with the patient and their family for this shift. This is harder than it seems. Checking out mentally is something we do 100's of times a day.

Don't believe it? How much do you know about your face book friends that you have never even met in person? Do you know as much about your own family?

Stay off of Face book and email and actually be present with this human that has entrusted you with their life. Did you hear that? Entrusted you...wow, how cool is that?!

Pay attention to how you feel. After you have done this a couple of times you will start to notice that you feel more connected to your job, it will start to feel alive.

Once you get to a place where you can 'feel' your practice you will be able understand easily why your practice needs to reflect your values.

Take the next step by noticing what things make you nuts throughout the shift.

What behaviors' in other nurses, patient's or families make you want to slit your wrists? Notice and then ask yourself if you are guilty of those same things. Maybe these are character traits you view as weak or needy. Do they make you nuts because they reflect a piece of you that you are trying to ignore or is it just plain ole annoying?

An example: One shift a patient's family was lamenting about the impending death of their loved-one. We were going to extreme measures to keep them living at that time. As this elderly patients family went on-and-on debating the withdrawal of care, one of them happened to speak up while I was in the room providing care. He said, 'If God had wanted mama to come home to Him He would have taken her already this morning in the ER. I think we have to fight to keep her alive the way God has fought to keep her alive.'

So, yea, this pushed many buttons inside me that I had no idea existed. I knew from the passionate ass-chewing I refrained from but wanted to give them that I needed to deal with it quickly. They pushed the button inside me that says, BE KIND FIRST. It is the non-negotiable for me in my practice. I didn't feel they were being very kind to mama. I wanted to respond to this family that God had already tried to take her home and that it was man that had intervened and saved her; not God. I wanted to remind them that the procedures we were performing were probably painful (not kind). I was annoyed beyond belief by the focus on how they needed to help God(as if God need help) rather than anyone worrying about how much pain mama was going through or what mama might want for her own life or how God had intended for her natural death to be before they intervened with a trip to ER.

Instead of allowing my inner patient pit-bull to emerge, I quickly finished care and got out of the room before my head exploded. I got a little angry that day and dare I say, a bit self-righteous with it.

It was really none of my business to judge or have an opinion about in the place. All I could do was to be kind to them in that moment and know they were dealing g with it as best they could in that moment.

Point is these were my own biases, pain points + prejudices to work out. Do you have a sense of your own yet?

Once you know what pushes your buttons you can soften your attitude and in the process learn what is important to you. Maybe your aggravation is just a signal you're letting go of one of your core beliefs about your practice. Or maybe it is just the way your body/mind/soul sends you the signal when it is full? Again pay attention for a few days and be honest with yourself about how you are feeling.

You have probably thought about this stuff in a broad sense without giving much thought to the detail.

It may be all you can do to keep floating in the first few months with the basics of daily job tasks. I get that. No worries. Come back here when you feel less overwhelmed and read this chapter again.

Get detailed and freakishly honest here. Get a poster board

and put it on your wall...then write out the answers to the following questions as you discover them. (**Note to Self:** this does not happen all at once.)

- Why are you a nurse?
- Do you view yourself as a healer or just a nurse?
- What part of this job lights your soul on fire?
- Are you concerned about your patient mind, body + spirit?
- What parts of your non-nursing life are important to you? Do you see any areas here that have changed recently?
- What types of patient situations leave you feeling empty?
- Are you feeling ambivalent about work? **Note to Self**: This could be a sign that you are overloaded and need to circle back to self care.
- What situations leave you feeling judgmental or hostile towards patients?
- What bias do you hold?
- What assumptions do you practice with now?
- What do you have that no one else has to give?(**Note to Self:** this is your unique medicine that is part of the purpose of your nursing career at a soul level.) It is stuff that is yours alone to give to the world.

What attitude or commitment is most important to you in your practice.

What is non-negotiable?

Now you are going to use those answers to start to craft your practice!

Yea, baby! These questions will not get answered in the span of one day. Understand that it may take closer to a year for you to understand it all. Some of the questions will make no sense whatsoever at this point in your awesome new career and that is okay. At some point there will something that happens in you shift that causes you to remember the question. That is the time to come back and answer it.

Define non-negotiable in your life + practice.

_____
_____
_____
_____

Nursing is intended to be an expression of the divine within you that nurtures that space within others. How do you think that can best be expressed?

_____
_____
_____
_____

Can you see a divine spark in what you do?

_____
_____
_____
_____

As your shifts pass this first year explore these things:

_____
_____
_____
_____

What is important to you?

_____
_____
_____
_____

What do you want your patient to feel from you as you nurse?

_____

_____

_____

_____

What values are important to you?

_____

_____

_____

_____

How can you infuse those into you practice?

_____

_____

_____

_____

How can you meet your patient where they are + respect that space?

_____

_____

_____

_____

What are you devoted to in your outside life?

_____

_____

_____

_____

Do you see that reflecting in your nursing?

_____

_____

_____

_____

What traits do you value in other nurses?

_____

_____

_____

_____

List some small adjustments you could make that would lift the entire vibe of your shift.

_____

_____

_____

_____

What do I want my patients to think, feel and KNOW about me at the end of my shift?

_____

_____

_____

_____

What feeling do I want to go home with at the end of every shift?

_____

_____

_____

_____

What feeling do you want to have at the end of your career?

_____

_____

_____

_____

If it was my parent or child what would I value as a good care?

_____
_____
_____
_____

Come back to this chapter once you have spent a few months in your practice. Then, just start to ask yourself these questions one at a time during your shift. Jot down notes on the back of your patient reports about how particular patients affected you. Go slow but go. I want you to have an ass-kicking practice that extends all your best parts in the world. I want you to be happy.

I practice these things every single shift. I could attempt to explain how transformational it is to set intention and infuse yourself into your practice and how these really simple questions help; it is just something you have to experience.

I promise though, once you can get there, this simple act changes things.

Focus Point: Your practice is a living thing and requires your devotion to flourish.

Action Step: Write down what you consider your best parts and start to think about how you can infuse these into your practice.

Mantra Mojo: *I will use my power for good.*

Tell me some ways that right here + right now you can use your power for good, Nurse Awesome. Free form style:

SACRED SPACE

The work you are doing on the planet, this whole nursing

thing? It is sacred work. The space you create with your

patient in the moments they trust

you with their life? It is sacred space. It is super-hard to

believe this about your new career while you are
in the middle of some of those crazy, out of control, oh my
god I can't believe I did this to myself shifts you will have as
you get adjusted to your new world.

It is no less true. The work you do is sacred work and it

happens in sacred space. You can use this profession as a

vehicle to express the highest and

best parts of who you are; or not.

You can let this 'job' become an act of worship; a devotion to
the divine spark within you; or not. I know there can be a lot
of 'junk' around the word 'sacred' and

'divine'. I ask that you not get all heady and over think it; no

need for all that stuff. Suspend your current thoughts

surrounding these words. Baggage down for a moment

please+ understand... This concept of sacred, it is not just a

God thing.

Webster's defines 'sacred' as:

- highly valued and important, deserving honor and respect
- set apart for the service or worship of something
- devoted exclusively to one service
- entitled to reverence and respect
- not to be violated, criticized, or tampered with

Your career and the relationships you create with your patients meet the criteria above, right? So yes, your practice is sacred.

I have been through some crazy experiences in my short time as a nurse. Some of those could have led me to a place where my practice had little, if any, connection to my heart. It is absolute survival to practice this way; closed up, just the facts, no personal connection to the patient.

At some point you are going to feel the missing piece.

Instead wondering what on earth has happened to the career you dreamt about like you did when hard stuff first popped up for you as a new nurse, you are going to think to yourself, 'I know this is not all there is to nursing.'

When you get here you'll know it is time to take your practice to a deeper level.

A place where human touches human and the sacred occurs.

Let me just be frank with you here. Some days the suffering and inhumanity you step into the middle are so offensive that you must operate from a space that remains far away from your heart.

Some days you will start out open and willing to meet your

patients in a sacred space only to find that some 'thing' sends you running back to the outskirts of that place.

People can and will do horrific things to themselves and each other. They may even try to hand some of that over to you by monopolizing your time, belligerent behavior, refusal to follow doctor's orders and flat out doing the opposite of what you ask.
You do not have to take any of that anger bullshit from them.

You do not have to let their nonsense make you angry.

You do not have to let their projection of fear leave you frustrated or wishing that you had a different assignment.

Chances are, especially as a new nurse that you will.

You may start the shift with the intention of being open with your patient only to find yourself thinking or saying some pretty hateful and judgmental things about your patient or their family before the day is done.

Don't throw stones at yourself or let those smarmy thoughts in your head make you decide that you are a horrible person or a crappy nurse. Not true. You are coping as well as you can with the tools you have at that moment.

So is your patient.

Most days, I remain open and allow my heart and head to guide me in equal parts. I say 'most' because there are days when no matter what I do to try and flip my attitude towards them the best I can do is to be polite to them and make sure they have their meds on time.

I had a patient not long ago that pulled the BiPAP off every time I left the room then claimed she did not know how it got removed. I get she was lonely and wanted company. I spent an hour in her room chatting thinking this would help however; there was nothing gonna fill the well of fear inside her that night. I sat right in front of her room to prove she was safe; no matter. That mask came off over and over. She would push the call light before I even got out of her room. I told her I would be back in 30 minutes and was monitoring her from the desk and not to worry. Nothing mattered. The moment she told me I was not meeting her needs I damn near snapped. Instead, I quietly (kind is important to me) asked her if she was ready to die? Of course, she told me no. I then explained to her that the mask was life support at this point in time and that if she removed it trying to get my attention and I was in another room then she would stop living. I told her that if this is how she felt I would call her son and daughter and ask them to come as we removed her mask so she would not be alone when she died. I told her that her actions were sending the clear message that she was ready to die. She was a bit shocked at my words however; she stopped ringing the call bell like it was a toy. I was kind and brutally honest with her and I viewed that space as sacred. It was probably not the kindest thing to do; I needed to get her attention though. I did.

Mean or needy people suck and can suck the life right out of you.

I make an effort to remain open because it is important to me and because I am firmly convinced that my nursing practice is the perfect vehicle for divinity to be expressed; even when I feel like hell.

This is no small statement to make.

'Even while' I feel like hell...hmmm

I believe that all of my life experience combines with my unique view on the world and my giant heart to help me be a vehicle for that sacred connection. I try to stay open to that connection.

It doesn't mean I never feel pissed off at my patient assignment. It does not mean that I go around talking to people about God or faith or Buddha or what they believe might happen when they die, or what meaning their life holds or any other of those highly-charged topics.

It simply means that I let Creator work through me for whatever conversation is in the highest good of my patient. Sometimes it is that heavy stuff, other times it is basic chatter while still other times it is hard core truth..

Believing that the time with my patient is sacred space might seem a bit odd however; it is what helps me stay balanced and keeps me from losing my shit on many a crazy night on the unit.

It helps me create meaningful work.

Have you ever considered your nursing practice to be something sacred? If you allowed yourself to think of your nursing practice as a direct expression of your personal belief system how would it change?

Would you still look at the mundane tasks you have to perform as a drag or would you consider every single thing you do to be divinely led?

You know that the work you do matters; to your family, to your patients and even to the world, right?

Do you know that the way you do that work matters, too?

It might feel like a stretch to think about sacred within all the 'stuff' that has to get done each shift. Getting meds from the Pyxis, changing linens, helping to the bathroom; all of those seem about as disconnected as you can get from anything remotely divine.

At least on the surface it does. It will be that way for awhile, sweetness, and that is okay. Divinity is never pushy or impatient so you should not get impatient or pushy with yourself to try and 'get' to this place in your practice either.

Just keep asking to find + connect with the sacred in all those seemingly mindless things and soon even something as simple as a pillow flip will feel like church.

Ask to be fully present. Ask to be beneficial and trust your gut to help you to that place.

Case in point for me:

I was in the room of an incredibly sick patient. They had come down from the floor on a rapid response call with issues oxygenating. There was some thought that they may be merely anxious but a high temp and heart rate pointed somewhere else so they got to come see us in the ICU at 1 am that shift.

When I introduced myself they were fighting hard to breathe with a BP in the tank. The phenoms of my unit and I were busy doing the million and one tasks that needed to all be done RIGHT NOW to help stabilize this patient. They were about to buy a vent and as I worked to prepare for that event I could not help but notice the 'deer in the headlights' look on the face of my patient. It was breaking my heart. They were obviously scared so I stopped what I was doing for a moment and touched their arm, looked at them in the eye, told them that while they were quite sick we were taking great care of them and then I asked if they had any questions about what was happening. Turns out they did so I answered them and went about my tasks. I was about to race out of the room when I noticed that they were sweating so much that their pillow had become soaked, it did not look comfy. So, I put my stuff in my pockets and again looked at them in the eye, asked them to lift their head and flipped their pillow over to the non-wet side. As I did this I said simply, 'you are not alone.'

It was a simple gesture at the time and honestly not something I connected to anything I would later call 'sacred work.'
Once the patient recovered they told their family that the only thing they remembered from the night was how scared they were and how 'this one nurse' took the time to make them comfortable and answer questions and how that simple act had made such a huge impact for them. The family relayed that they felt valued, like a person not a disease and that they felt safe in my care because I was looking at even their smallest needs being met.

I never thought a pillow flip could be so important. To know that a simple act like that could communicate that this person mattered to me and that they were safe, well, that floored me.

It also defined sacred space to me. I'd been noticing how much good-work, soul-work could be done in the small encounters between patient and nurse for a while. This exchange really drove the point home for me.

I used to think the only parts of my job that mattered were the big things. You know, noticing a blood pressure or heart rate change and taking steps to correct it, looking for the subtle signs that something bad was about to happen for them and heading that bad off at the pass. Those things were really in the front of my vision of what it meant to be a great nurse.

Now I believe that noticing they have a dry mouth and offering a swab when they are NPO or offering to help them wash their face, braid their hair, flip the pillow to the cool side, well, all of these things are just as important in the 'great nurse' definition.

My patients need to know through everything I do that they matter.

For me it translates to this You matter, you are safe=presence of divinity=sacred space.

Look for these types of experiences in your own shifts. Use the tools in this book to bridge the gaps in your practice until you can get your bearings about you enough to look for these pieces. You might just revisit this chapter 6 months from now.

It can help you define your personal 'why' and lead you to more fulfilling shifts more quickly and on a more regular basis.

The extra energy you create for yourself when you get here is worth the gas it took to get there.

Focus Point: Finding the place where your sacred lives is a game-changer. It is the difference between the guitar solo in your favorite song being played with or without the amplifier. They are both okay but one is communicated much more powerfully than the other, right?

Action Step: Begin to consider the possibility that your work is sacred. As new as you are to this place consider that you are a vehicle for sacred stuff!

Mantra Mojo: My work is an expression of divinity through me. I am honored to hold this sacred space.

Dear Registered Nurse Awesome-

It seemed to have snuck up on you, huh?
Suddenly you are not a student anymore and
there is a lot that is riding on your choices.

Don't let it overwhelm you, okay? You really
are prepared for it. You really are a great
nurse.

Stop and ask questions when you need.
Remember that you have a ton of knowledge in
you already. No instructor to get permission from
now.

It is just you⋯but you are never really all alone⋯

Yay Team Awesome!

THE ROUGH DAYS

It's both challenging + interesting as a new nurse in the ICU.

Though, I imagine any area in nursing is like that these first 30 days.

In my world, beeps + buzzes come at me from all conceivable directions. It is intimidating to most of us by the days end so I can only imagine how it is for my patients and their families.

I swear, by the end of a 12-hour shift my brain aches for the solitude of my car. The complex equipment and invasive monitoring, the suffering, the lengths we go to in order to heal?

These are things I didn't really think about in nursing school.

Of course, I 'knew' that all of this happened. I had seen it to some extent. I just never expected it to hit me so hard. I did not grasp the implications of causing harm in order to heal.

I never expected to wear the suffering of the folks I take care of home with me.

It happens more than I would like though.

HIPAA prevents me from sharing most of what happens on a typical day. Pay attention to what is happening around you and you will find your own stories to demonstrate this point; we cause harm to heal.

My heart breaks for each of my patients + their families. Loads of stress accompanies the phrase 'Intensive Care Unit.' I do not know these people yet still, I feel connected to them in a way difficult to put in words.

I cry with them, for them and over the pain they must endure. I am even known to tear up giving report to the next shift as I relay the pain I am sure they must be going through.
I am changed by my experience of caring for them.

I am told that will fade away and eventually I will not even remember the name let alone the face or the medical issue of a patient. I am told that this type of callousness is something that I 'need' to develop in order to survive in the world of nursing.

I hope not.

I have found a way to 'let it go' and not take on the suffering of others however; I have not yet reached the place where I am disconnected from the human-ness of the people I care for each shift.

My hope is that by consciously creating a practice that honors the sacred space I share with my patient that I will always see humanity.

It's my intent to never get to that disconnected place.

When I first started nursing, my mission was simple. I wanted to heal everyone in my care, period. Yes, I am aware that this sounds irrational and unlikely yet, I was certain I would witness broken souls rise up and leave the confines of their illness every day.

Some days that happens and some days healing takes the form of death rather than life.

I believe the human spirit is resilient and that has been

proven to me over and over as people I just 'knew' could not survive their illness have left the unit. There have been others I never expected to go downhill that do exactly that; and rather quickly I might add.

One of things you will be forced into doing these first few months is to take a closer look at your own beliefs about death and dying. These are two different things, you know? No matter where you work in the hospital system, you have to do that in order to survive what you witness. It helps you makes sense of things, make peace with things, be able to more quickly sort and process what you will see on some of the rougher days as a new nurse.

I've always believed that positive thoughts + positive energy are healing. I believe in the power of humans to release things that are weighing them down in illness and that has not changed for me.

What has changed is this simple truth: healing is different for everyone.

For some, healing is indeed getting up and out of bed and back to life as it was before their illness. For others, it is learning how to just get back to living; no matter how many adjustments are needed because of their illness.

For even more people healing is something even simpler.

For some, healing is just a few more months with their beloved.

For some it is seeing a kid get married, graduate from school or reach some other milestone.

For others it is as simple as petting their dog or hugging the adult child they haven't seen in years one more time before they die.

As hard as it was for me to accept as a new nurse, the truth of the matter is that often times healing only comes with death.

You may find in these first few months that there is an odd kind of guilt you carry when a patient dies. It might show up for you as self-doubt, as if you did not do 'enough' to help them keep living.

Your rational mind will tell you the truth; you didn't cause the illness nor can you cure the illness. Everyone dies; you are not in control...blah, blah, blah.
I am aware that it seems fairly ridiculous to feel like you could have changed the outcome for a patient and it took me a while to figure out why it was happening for me.

I am in the healing profession to heal. Death felt like failure to me. It felt like the worse possible outcome for my patient. It felt like it violated my prime directive as a nurse.

A few months in and my views started to shift. Now, I've seen a lot of death and dying.

Now, I know for a fact, via my own observations, that there are many things much worse than death.

Now, I embrace the simple truth that I cannot possibly know the plan of each soul while they are on this earth. I accept that death might be one part of a plan I cannot see nor understand.

How do you feel about death and dying; your own and that of those you are caring for at work each shift?

Is it different for you when the death is expected as

opposed to when it is not expected?

What will you say to the family of the decedent once it occurs?

Will you feel horrible about it? Will you know how to let it go?

How are you going to deal with it when a patient dies unexpectedly?

Have you thought about it in depth at all?

It will help if you take a second to answer those questions up front to the extent possible. Then, pay attention to how you feel once you are in that situation.
It helps me to I say this simple phrase as I walk past the ICU waiting area on the way in to the unit each day.

'Let me be a beneficial presence'

I have no idea what I will face for the night. I know that I do not get to choose how I nurse but that I can always choose how I nurse those souls.

A quick glance at the waiting room gives me hint of the night to come. Multiple small groups of crying people, well, that tells me this shift will most likely be filled with equal parts art and science behind this craft I have chosen.

I try to put myself into their place. I don't know them now but by the end of 12 hours I will know their stories, the way of their illness, the dance they have left in them, what they need to do to consider themselves healed from their illness.

I'll learn what they have given up and what they've fought to keep and I will learn oh so much about what they are afraid of leaving behind.

If I am lucky I hear the stories from the patient directly. More likely from the ICU bed it will be the family speaking on behalf of the loved one; half here and half among the dead.

Families love to talk about the illness so I make plans and scramble to catch up my charting so they can feel free to ramble; I think it helps them heal so I gladly go thru the extra effort.

They always remind me of my dad when he needed to speak to everyone and anyone about my mom's fight. To validate existence, to let everyone know how hard she tried to defeat the disease, to show people her strength when she 'appeared' weak.

Who knows the exact whys of it? I only know that there is transformative power in this place of sharing for your patient's kinfolk if you can allow it.

Don't let a busy shift rob them of the healing it provides.

They are just as much your patient as the one in the bed.

Many times I am left to interpret the stories from the scars + lines their bodies show to me as I am caring for them or a family members remembrance of the person they were 'before'.

The most awesome nights for me are the ones when my patient can actually talk to me, no matter how hard it is to hear what they have to say. I take the time to listen and am invariably enriched by it.

No matter how busy, I always ask what brings them joy, what thing they love and what they want their life to be about and no matter how sick they are I always, always, always tell them that they matter.

I spent a whole semester learning about 'transition to professional nursing practice' and not once did we chat about how to handle my own emotions as I watched a person take their last breath.

No professor ever told me that my simple presence mattered as much as my knowledge of their disease.

I thought it was all about the pathophys and the cure, you know?

Not one person told me that there would be many, many days I would wonder what the hell I had gotten myself into and they certainly never mentioned that I would want to quit before the first month was out.

No one shared how to find myself and truly let my own unique perspective on the world shine thru my work.
In all my time in school not one person ever said the word sacred yet as I have walked through the first few years of my nursing career I am hard pressed to find any piece of this work that is not sacred.

There will be days when you seem to have forgotten basic nursing concepts and others you whip through your skills with ease. Lots of days you stammer through teary-eyed + worried that nothing you do will matter, some days you will leave not caring if it matters or not.

Sometime in the middle of a seemingly perfect shift a particularly tough patient situation will remind you of your own mortality or how precious your child is to you or how much you miss someone you love.

Being human connects us.

We see ourselves in others. This is exactly as it should be.

There will rough days. They didn't talk about them much in school because no adjective is accurate for how they make you feel inside.

They didn't waste theory time giving you pointers because we all have to feel our way though these spaces leaning on our own faith + understanding.

They don't show you any 'how-to's' because no matter the try, each rough spot is unique and stands on its own without a manual or guide to get through it. These are times when only an open heart can guide you and other times your heart will close up simply because it cannot bare the pain of what it is witnessing.

I am one of those annoying people that find the rainbow within every rainstorm however; I have not meant to sugar coat anything here.
If you have made it to the end of this book I know you are fully schooled in the potholes no one pointed out to me as I made my way into the world as a brand new nurse.

This first year, it is a dose of reality that few of us 'newbies' are prepared for really.

Focus Point: There is not a tried and true formula that gets you through all of it this first year. The best thing is to lean on your training and listen to your heart. Ask for help when you need it but know that you already know a lot of stuff, Nurse Awesome. Somewhere along the way the connection to your craft will marry both the art and science of nursing and your sacred space will emerge. It will be unique; like you. Time goes by quickly and you will get through it as a thriving and passionate nurse and you will be a beneficial presence, no doubt!

Action Step: Take a break when you have a rough day. You don't have to be tough all the time.

Mantra Mojo: *I am a beneficial presence. I am strong and capable and loving and brave and I have all that I need to be an awesome nurse.*

You will be shocked at how much you still have to learn when you start your first job as a nurse

Be kind to yourself as you learn. This is called a nursing practice not a nursing perfect.

If you start feeling like the shift, the charge nurse, the world is out to get you stop and check your own attitude. Most of what happens outside of us is just a reflection of what is happening inside us. If your cup is full then it is up to you to empty it.

If all else fails, go back to the basics of your practice. When you are losing your shit, think safety and everything will be okay.

POTHOLES TO POSSIBILITIES

A great friend of mine that listened to me whine the first 30 days of my nursing career asked me casually one day why on earth I decided to be a nurse if it was such a pain in the ass.

It's not all bad, although I imagine from her non-nursing perspective seeing me in tears one minute and with my head in my hands the next, well, it probably looked like it was a huge pain in the ass.

The fact is that nursing is a career that takes you to the extremes in human emotion; both your patients and your own. That can suck the life out of you at times.

It will test everything you think you know about people and life and reveal things to you that you never even thought were inside you, or inside other humans for that matter.

Nursing requires you bring your A-game every single day. There are many possibilities for deep and meaningful connection with humans. Witnessing suffering + tragic stuff, well, that will sure enough help you get in touch with the spark of divinity that lives within you and cause you to appreciate your life.

So, there is a horrible side to being a nurse.

Potholes exist, yea, but so do possibilities. Which you see depends solely on you. Just like all of your life, your focus is something you alone govern. So in the middle of JCAHO and your management team and all the crazy-ass stuff happening around you; the way you nurse is your choice. Always and your choice alone.

That kicks 1000 kinds of ass, huh?

While the gritty parts of this profession may leave you head in hands and filled with tears from time-to-time, those tears are the perfect vehicle for traveling to some of the most amazing places.

It is easy to close up when things get crazy on your shift. It is easy to let the wheels come off our spirit when we hit the potholes.

If you can focus on no other thing when you hit those potholes I want you to think this, 'This is merely an opportunity for me to connect with the divine and express that through my nursing.'

In all honesty, when you are knee-deep in GI bleed feeling 'divine' or connected to sacred will be no where on your radar. The only connection you may feel to sacred in the middle of a code is your own plea to God to help your patient live.

You will be in full-on survival mode in those moments and that is okay. I am not suggesting you will always love every aspect of your work here. I am telling you that you can marry the whole of it together into something extraordinarily awesome.

I am telling you that all pieces of it carry connection to divinity. All.

I am telling you that if you spend time getting rooted in the things that are important to you in your practice, if you take some time and become devoted, if you release negativity before it builds up and starts to weigh you down then even the tough times begin to look not so tough.

Honestly.

Do you know why you love nursing? Take a minute and write those reasons down in your nursing bible book. You may want to refer to them from time-to-time.

Here is my list. I bet there are at least a few things we agree on here.

- It's fast-paced + you never stop learning.
- It allows me to do honest, hard work each day that, at the end of the day, makes me feel like my efforts actually mattered.
- It allows me to do work I believe matters.
- I love that I can be kind without being questioned. I feel great at the end of the day. I am often exhausted however; I am always filled up, feeling blessed and thankful for my own life-it centers me.
- I love that I see something different everyday-I am never bored and I am always learning new things.
- I love that my experience and knowledge are doing something of actual value
- It allows me to reaffirm the things I believe in
- I love seeing other people smile, and mean it...I love the way the universe puts me in hard places and brings me through them with my patients
- It allows me to be an ear for other peoples suffering-I am able to listen to what is 'ailing' them-sometimes that is just body but most of the time people open up about what is emotionally ailing them
- It puts me in a place where I must practice patience and ask for help to provide the best care
- I love that I can smile and be genuine, use my heart and be caring and that this is actually something that is appreciated by patients rather than stomped on by corporate mucky mucks.
- It jazzes me to see people get it or begin to take

ownership over their health and connect the dots of how their actions affect their lives.

- o I am energized into wanting to teach people that they can have some control over their own stuff, what they focus on they bring to them, what they think about they expand, if they put good out they get good back.

This is a running list that grows larger and more filled with love as I gain experience in this field.

Most days that is, some days I am running full throttle from the moment I walk in to the moment I leave and it feels like just when I think the shift could not get any harder, it does.

No lie on those days I am hard pressed to come up with a couple of bullet points to love up this profession.

I s'pect this will be the way for you, too. You'll learn to go with the flow of things, to appreciate the good days + the bad days without partiality to either.

Paying some attention to your heart/mind/spirit will help you get in your groove more quickly.

When I get down to the end of it all, I know, that the real reason I started nursing was to help end suffering by sharing kindness + joy. I want to be a beneficial presence.

Yea, big statement there, I know. It sounds lofty to some and I have been called any number of variations of crazy for even having this thought; I don't mind it much.

I don't believe suffering is needed in this world or this profession.

I believe it is optional not mandatory to let fear work in your life.

I believe that every moment of our life we can choose to express joy.

I wrote this book because I want the same things for you. I know that you can feel joyful on this journey and that suffering as you move from student nurse to registered nurse is not mandatory.

You are going to fall into a few piles of suck as you get adjusted and since I fell into them before you I figured I should put up some 'caution-this thing sucks' signs along your path.

At the end of the day, nursing makes me feel like I am living with my heart fully engage in humanity and giving the best of myself each day.

On the hardest of days I remember that my presence can be beneficial; or not. I know that I get to choose my focus regardless of what is happening.

I hope this book has helped you know that you don't have to suffer. It is sometimes super-tough to be a nurse. The transition to practice is no better or worse; it is just filled with things that look big and scary because you have never been a nurse before.

You have what it takes to be awesome even in this first year of practice so don't spend time beating yourself or engaged in unhelpful practices because it is tough. It is not helpful.

Instead, see if you can spend time discovering how to craft your own practice in order to bring the shiniest parts of your soul to the profession rather than losing your shit. Some days you will dig the hell out of what you do and others you will be scratching your head wondering what on earth you can do to get out of this place. No matter how much you 'love' nursing you WILL have days that you want to run as far away from this profession as you can run.

You will find a balance between them soon enough.

Nursing really is all the good + bad of human existence rolled into a single job description. Nothing else is really like it.

Once you figure this out you will feel supercharged by your superhero-like ability 'to nurse'.

Sometime during this first year you will realize you cannot truly nurse a patient to the best of your ability until you have learned to first nourish yourself. This is a wholly empowering place. Be as gentle with yourself as you are with patients until you get there.

Remember, it is your practice not your perfect.

It has been an honor to share this part of your journey with you. I truly appreciate your presence here + hope these words have been a beneficial presence.

The Nurse Awesome Nation needs your heart and soul to change our culture; I look forward to meeting you there.

Tools to AMP up Your Awesome!

So use the stuff on the pages that follow however you feel is best for you. There is not a right or wrong way. No grading will be done, you cannot fail.

Just have fun with them and enjoy the experience of being a new nurse!

Here is a list of the things that follow.

- Finding Your Mojo
- Down and Dirty Plan to Maintain Sanity
- Chapter 3 Implementation Plan Companion
- Morning Magics
- End of Shift Magic
- Love Note Magic
- Signs + Symptoms of an Overloaded Nurse
- The Aftermath of Fear: Expansion vs. Contraction
- Empty Your Cup
- What-If's
- Prayer to Dissolve Fear
- Building Trust
- Examine Your Bias
- Love Letters to Awesome Nurses
- Love Letter to My Patient

Finding Your Mojo

The end of this book is really just a new place to start.

We have looked at the rough days that will come up as you start your new career.

We have learned a few ways to disengage from that rough stuff so that you can have some sort of life that is not surrounded by the suffering.

We touched on how to keep yourself calm and peaceful so that you do not become bitter and jaded before the year is out.

We have dipped our toe in the deep end of the pool by considering your nursing career as a direct extension of you.

This is where you find your mojo. You know, your magic power? The thing you have that no one else could possibly ever have. The medicine that you have to give to the world.

That stuff, yes...THAT stuff!

Once you find it you will start to truly shift your focus. You will see your nursing practice as an absolute art form. You will see it as something within your complete control.

You will see yourself as an artist and your nursing practice as your palette. See, your nursing practice is the chance for your to show the world how you feel, who you are, how you believe human kind to be and what you believe to be most important.

You are probably thinking big-whoop, right? So you know all of these things, you take the time to craft your practice, you get in touch with your mojo and all that stuff. How does any of that make a difference in the time you spend running around nursing people for 12 hours a day?

Connecting to your magic allows you to consciously put your unique medicine into the world.

This place of resonance, where your magic is, where you know that you bring something special to this party.

It allows things to change.

It allows you to remain balanced when chaos happens around you.

It allows you to feel you are doing work that matters because that work is an expression of you.

It allows you to view your work as connection to the Divine.

It allows you to determine the non-negotiable things you want to express.

It changes everything in your practice and in your life.

Your magic and your devotion to it are what bind all the pieced together. None of it is useful alone however; when you start to see them as part of a great story, as part of your reason for being...well, that is when things get super-charged.

Your magic is your medicine and since I have dropped enough hints through this text. I may as well come right out and tell you. Your practice isn't something that you do, Nurse Awesome. It is something that you are..a living extension of you in the world. While it is always inside you, you have to do the work to find it. You are worth the effort!

Down-n-Dirty Plan to Maintain Sanity

If you do nothing else that this book mentions you will see some shift toward the positive if do these things, sweetpea.

- Do not catastrophize; nothing is as bad as it seems
- Stay in the present moment; don't dwell on past screw ups or perceived inadequacy
- Pay attention to your hesitations; these tell you were you need to gain confidence ONLY, they are not indicators that you suck
- Find a mentor on your floor, someone other than your preceptor, preferably someone that approaches nursing the way you approach it. In other words, if you are a smart ass then you probably shouldn't buddy up with a non smarty pants person, ya know?
- Write down what you don't get each shift and go home and look it up, then study that shit until you do get it.

CHAPTER 3 IMPLEMENTATION PLAN

Wow, the first month went by fast! I am starting to get my feet under me a bit. Let me learn these things to help my new-self not feel so damn new. My awesomeness will shine thru a bit more clearly in my performance as a nurse if I take some time and figure out these things:

The crash cart is located:

_____

_____

_____

The items I always make sure are in my room are:

_____

_____

_____

The items I always make sure are in my pockets are:

_____

_____

_____

The skills I am confident performing are: The skills I want to work on are:

_____

_____

_____

Equipment on my floor I have no idea how to operate:

_____

_____

_____

The nurse rock star that is going to help me learn that equipment's location and how to use it is?

_____
_____
_____

How do we admit patient to this floor?

_____
_____
_____

Are there some JCAHO things I need to always do in the chart?

_____
_____
_____

Psychosocial Situations I encountered this week:

_____
_____
_____

Psychosocial situations I need some help navigating through:

_____
_____
_____

What procedures so I need to make sure I learn about this month?

_____
_____
_____

What lab values am I sketchy on?

_____
_____
_____

What medications am I going to see frequently on this floor?

_____

_____

_____

What doctors usually admit to this floor?

_____

_____

_____

What standing orders exist for this floor?

_____

_____

_____

What will I do when there is an emergency?

_____

_____

_____

Three things I will I do when I feel stupid.

_____

_____

_____

Three things I will do when I feel scared.

_____

_____

_____

MORNING MAGICS

Start your day or your shift with a simple prayer or ask.

It sets your intention on having a beneficial day; to all people involved. (ps, you don't have to use mine, make up one of your own if you like)

Make me an instrument of peace and healing today

Allow me to stay balanced and calm in crisis

Allow me to stay patient when things get off track

Allow me to remain open in times of fear

Allow me to bring hope where there is none

Allow me to dispense my unique medicine freely so all may use it as needed

Allow me to be a beneficial presence

END OF SHIFT MAGIC

End your day or your shift with a bit of thanks or gratefulness and release of all people involved. I do this on the way to get my stuff before I even clock out (again, you don't have to use mine, make up one of your own if you like)

Thank you for allowing me to bring peace and healing to my patients Thank you for allowing me to stay focused during crisis Thank you for helping me stay calm when I was afraid Thank you for guidance as I use my unique medicine I release all emotions that I may be carrying that belong to others I trust my patients highest and best good is being done Thank you for helping me a beneficial presence

LOVE NOTE MAGIC

No template needed here, loves. Grab a glitterful notebook from the store, fancy moleskin, colorful construction paper-whatever you like. Just dedicate that book/space for telling YOU how amazing YOU are..Seriously...try it for 10 days and you will see your whole demeanor change.

They do not have to be long or extravagant or perfect. No one will see them but you. Some of my pages are filled with long detailed buckets of love to me while others are just a few words scribbled in crayon. Each one has this in common; they help me focus on the great stuff inside me and in doing that they help me get through the tougher things. They keep me expanding in the direction I choose to go rather, where I place my intent, rather than just following the trail of negativity that a string of crappy shifts can lead me down.

For every one thing that 'might' not work out the way you intended through you day as a nurse there are at least 5 more that work out amazingly well. Remind yourself of these things.

I know it seems odd at first to tell yourself how awesome you are..writing in the third person can make you feel strange. Just do it anyway. Okay?

There is some powerful magic in consciously reminding yourself that you are incredible.

SIGNS + SYMPTOMS OF AN OVERLOADED NURSE

This happens to all of us from time-to-time. We get so engaged in meeting the needs of other people that we totally forget ourselves.

No worries, you can fix this with some self-directed TLC.

First though, know that if you get in the habit early on in your career of making time to disengage and reframe your day every day then you will not find yourself in this place quite as often.

Take the presence of these things on a more than a one day/week basis as a whisper from your body, heart and mind that you need a breather. Pay attention or they will start to holler at you. Not fun!

S+S that signal a need for TLC:

- Oversensitivity
- Mood Swings/Irritability/Restlessness
- Excessive Anger or Anxiety for no reason you can pinpoint
- Inability to focus and memory issues
- Muscle tension and sleepless nights
- Taking lots of sick days or feeling of dread going to work
- Increase in headaches or stomach issues
- Apathy where you once felt engaged and joyful

These are just a few things you might notice. If you see any of them start to creep into your life change something, pronto!

It might even help to make a pact with a nurse buddy that you will check in with each other once a week just for the purpose of gauging where your attitude lies. This is self-care 101-you must do this to keep nursing for years to come!

The thing about PTSD is that it can sneak up on you. You are just moving along in your day-to-day as a nurse when suddenly you notice that you are not so on fire about this career anymore.

It may show up as a feeling in your gut that something is just not 'right'. Listen to your gut.

Don't be that nurse that ignores her own body, mind and spirit and ends up in the bed as a result of some stress-related PTSD-ish thing that could have been redirected if you had been paying attention to yourself.

We need your light so please pay attention!

THE AFTERMATH OF FEAR
EXPANSION VS. CONTRACTION

I can always tell when I am afraid because I start procrastinating like crazy. For example, I finished this book 4 months ago and promptly found a lot of reasons not to finish it. No matter how cleverly I disguised the reasons they were all just me being afraid I had nothing of value to offer you + that my experience was not worth anything.

That procrastination bleeds over into all areas of life. It makes me super-shaky about all my actions; it makes me question everything from a place in my where the underlying feeling is

"Hey Melissa, you shouldn't do that because you are gonna suck"

It makes me hesitate. It closes me up to solutions, to moving forward, to trusting myself, to taking definitive action quickly.

Many of my friends call this my 'smallness talking'

I have to agree...all of that is a fancy way to say it makes me contract. This is a crummy place to be in.

That is not what I want my life to be about.

So, while I cannot always come up with the label 'fear' for what I am feeling, I can always recognize it because it makes me feel small and less capable than I am.

I know how fear makes me feel: closed up

And I know how I feel when I am not afraid: Opened up

To me these are the most reliable measure.

Do you know how fear shows up for you in your life?

If not, spend some time looking for clues to its presence. Is there something you want to do that you put off? Is there an activity that makes you weak in the knees to think about doing?

In nursing, fear shows up in all sorts of places and it is not something you want to make a part of your practice. It throws a pothole onto your path every day you allow it to close you up. It can cause hesitation where you need to act quickly.

Yes, it is inevitable this first year because you are going to be having experiences you have never had before. The unknown brings fear and with it many opportunities to expand or contract.

Learning how to quickly measure the validity of your fear will help you build a solid practice more quickly. It will help you choose expansion more quickly.

Releasing fear will help bring you balance into your personal life + it is the only way that you can show up fully for your patients.

Try using this simple tool to quickly check for fear during your day:

- Am I feeling peaceful and calm even though I am in the middle of a busy shift? If not, what emotion am I feeling?
- Allow for the possibility that your emotion is fear in disguise.
- Am I feeling overwhelmed with tasks?
- Am I putting off doing something that needs done?
- Am I worried about the outcome if I perform a task

- Do I need to perform a task I have never done or am uncomfortable performing?
- Does this fear serve me in this moment?
- Is the patient situation uncomfortable for me?
- Do I feel capable of providing competent care?
- Is my feeling illogical for the circumstance?

Once you start asking yourself these types of questions you start to get a handle on whether or not you should shift directions because of fear and get some help or if you can focus your effort on expanding through the fear without help. Patient safety is the common denominator here. Get help if you need it..period.

The next piece of this will take a while to figure out for yourself. There is no exact formula because we are all different.

It is mostly about you paying attention in your own life. Invest the time cause you are totally worth it.

Whatever it is you are going through based on the answers above, ask yourself these questions

Do I feel closed or open while in that space? Is it legit fear or made up fear? Does it make me open up to possibilities or stay closed to any possible solution or resolution?

Here is the thing..Your natural state of being is one of peacefulness, wellness and openness. Lots of stuff can happen in the day to make that shift into the land of fear.

Name some of those things here:

Some feelings that indicate for me I am in the thick of that small, closed up + contracted place:

- ➢ The jitters or butterflies in my tummy
- ➢ Excessive hunger(might be lack of appetite too)
- ➢ Sweating, increased heart rate or breathing shallow
- ➢ Putting off tasks or decisions
- ➢ Inability to make a choice
- ➢ Crankiness..When my patience is short

Any of those could be a clue telling you that you are closed up. This whole 'expansion vs. contraction philosophy' does not have to get fancy. Just recognize that when you are overloaded or afraid you close yourself up and cut yourself off from the flow of your life.
I call this getting out of my groove. It is super-simple to feel when that happens. It is a bit more difficult for me to actually admit to myself that I have allowed myself to get overloaded and actually do something about it.

Once you get clear on the simple fact that you allowed yourself to get overwhelmed by fear you can resolve it. Not before.

The best part is that in all the 'stuff' that will happen in your busy nursing life that you have o control over this is one area you get total control over from day one.

It feels awesome to know that you get to choose whether or not you want to reframe things in your brain and do anything different... If you have checked your baggage and you are not afraid then you might need to empty your cup...

EMPTY YOUR CUP

Getting rid of or 'dumping' all the emotion and stress that accumulates around you during your shift is super-important for your personal health and longevity in this career.

You will be riding a wave of positive emotion and excited energy as you emerge from school and enter your brand new career. Thankfully, it will carry you for a while through the tough things you will face. Not so good is that it might also make it seem like you don't need to empty your cup at all.

So think of this exercise as preventative medicine for your mind, body, spirit and heart. Your patients need you to stay amazing and shiny so that they can heal, besides, awesomeness like you should stay in top form emotionally, physically and mentally.

So pay attention to this area of your practice at the end of each shift by asking a simple question: How do I feel???

Stop and listen to the answer. Are you smiling at shift's end or dragging yourself to the car? The stuff junking up your spirit shows itself in lots of ways: the tension in your shoulders, the upset tummy, and crankiness, over or under eating, overreaction to small stressors, feeling miserable on your way into work. This could be a long list.

Listen rock star, your spirit only has these jacked up ways to get your attention and tell you it needs help to balance or unload all the strong emotions you keep gathering. It is up to you to pay attention.

If you get in the habit of emptying that cup early on and continue to practice 'emptying' then you are much less likely to suffer debilitating stress, PTSD, compassion fatigue etc. You are less likely to hate your job before the year is out.

This exercise is easy and surprisingly effective at setting you back to a clean slate. It empowers you to keep your own health in check. It shifts thinking quickly back to taking great care of you rather than being focused on the care of patients.

Do it at the end of each shift for best results, before you even turn on the car to head for home.

EMPTY YOUR CUP EXERCISE

Sit still for a moment...Get comfortable + take a deep breath in...

Imagine yourself standing at the center of a vast + lush green field

Release your breath as you become aware of your body and how it feels to move about the field..Notice any areas of tension in your body as you move about the vast + lush green field

Breathe in again and notice any heaviness you may feel as you move freely about the vast+ lush green field

As you continue to breathe in and out slowly you find yourself standing in the center of the field holding a large silver chalice.

It is large and it shines like the light of the sun. It is heavy and difficult to hold onto even while standing still. Carrying it any distance is impossible,.

As you look down into the chalice you notice it is filled with some sort of liquid, sloshing back + forth as you struggle to maintain your balance.

You immediately come to understand this liquid as the leftover parts of all the emotional and stressful events throughout the day,

You quickly come to know these liquid emotions do not belong to you and that there is no need to come to know them each personally'

You are free to release them. You do not need to carry them

any longer.

You take a big breath in and smile at the thought of the weight being gone. As you exhale you empty the contents of the silver chalice and notice as the vast + lush green field absorbs the all the liquid that was in your cup.

There is no more tension in your body, no more heaviness-you feel light and energized and can once again move about the vast + lush green field freely.

Your cup is empty.

Open your eyes and give thanks for the feeling of being fully empty

What If's

What if you find yourself lost in the world of what if?

What-if...You know this is just a phrase to by us time because our brain is scared of the consequence of the action, right?

What if you were certain of the outcome, how would it change things? Here is quick reframe...for those 2 little words...

" What-if" is quite the curious thing The power to halt
Before one step is braved
No matter the journey
6 small letters arranged by some other person To describe *their* fear Or perhaps *their* curiosity
That we claim as our own
We give it permission to halt our hopes Erase possibility
Quell uniqueness
Our hearts power given too easily to just two words

So... 'what-if' these small 6 letters **first** labeled an adventure of the most glorious kind Instead of the nightmare we so easily conjure.

Like so many other things we have twisted It keeps us still 'what-if'....Instead we said..'Why of course this will be easy' ...'Absolutely we can do this thing'...'No doubt it will all be okay' ...'Certainly I will succeed'
Without Its mystery perhaps we smile, look at our fear and say..

'what-if I move forward
anyway?'

PRAYER/REQUEST TO DISSOLVE FEAR

Allow me to be transparent with myself so that I may identify all the places fear stops me in my practice. Help me look at my fears as an opportunity for growth.

Help me lay my ego aside and ask for help. I know I am not my fear, so while I allow myself to feel them I will let them move through me without holding onto them for longer than needed.

I release them with ease and grace and welcome the state of balance that is naturally within me I trust that all is well in my world and my actions are divinely led.

BUILDING TRUST

In the time it takes to introduce yourself as the nurse for the shift you expect someone to trust you with their life. You don't have the same kinda time to build relationship like in the outside world.

Patients will trust you because they have no choice, really.

Think about that for a minute. Doesn't that give you goose bumps? We get to do that every single day that we nurse.

Awesome power, huh?

It's up to you not to break that trust. There is an easy way to do that, Nurse Awesome.

Do what you say you are going to do. Period.

Chose your actions carefully and your promises to your patient even more carefully.

Every time we miss the mark they take back a tiny piece of the trust they gave us at shift change. You are in charge.

Create a trusting space for your patients, please. Not only will it make your own job much easier it will pave a smooth path for every other healthcare professional that comes after you.

Be kind to all of us!

EXAMINE YOUR BIAS

It is not always easy to have patience with your patients.

Many factors go into the shift and sometimes, despite your best intentions, a patient will push your buttons in a way that makes it super-tough to be kind.

Even as awesome as you are, you will run into these. First off, know that it is okay that you are not always Susie Sunshine. No one can ALWAYS be upbeat.

Secondly, remember your out landscape reflects you inner landscape so if you are finding yourself a bit more edgy than your norm take a look at what is going on in your life. It is almost a sure bet that there is some part of YOU that you are neglecting that is making it difficult to fully invest in others.

My particular bias surrounds mean detoxers; regardless of the substance. When I get a patient like this my first reaction used to be a huge groan. Like, they did this to themselves and now I have to spend an entire shift being mistreated by them because they are angry at what they did!

I always have to work to be supportive of these folks. So my shift is just a constant stream of prayers. Now that I have my feet under me a bit I just take a deep breath and give a silent thanks because I know I am about to learn a lot about myself and the world and human behavior and pain and all the other jacked up things this gift comes disguised as for me. I also ask for as many angels as are available to come on around and help support me during my time with that person.

I make a point of spending some extra time with these folks at the start of the shift discussing their needs with them and trying to give them some control over the shift. I have been known to tell unruly people that they will have choices again once they go home but that while they are with me, in the ICU, their safety and wellbeing is my top priority, which means they may have to temporarily lose some of the freedom they enjoy at home. That seems to quiet them down.

Another tool I use is this simple checklist below. It sort of shifts me into the patients' shoes; which makes it easier to give great care when folks are challenging. Ask yourself these questions prior to caring for those tough ones!

What is the anger really about? ***Note to*** **Self**: it always involves fear!

- Have you made an effort to let them control their care?
- What is the support system this patient has at home?
- Is there some need that is not met that you can help with like food, warmth or toileting?
- Are you providing awesome care for them or avoiding them?
- Is there a medicinal assistant you need to use to ease their anxiety?

To soften me even more I ask these questions. I usually ask these questions regardless of the patient type. It helps me stay focused on being kind when things get super-busy on the unit.

- Would you want to be your patient?
- What kind of nursing care would make you feel empowered and like you had a tiny bit of control?
- How would you want to be spoken to?
- If it were me in the bed what would I need?

Love Letter to My Patient

Hello. Welcome to my world. I realize this stay is not something you are pleased about. I don't blame you. This is not your comfort zone and your outside life can't be put on hold for you.

Being a patient can be a bit frustrating and confusing. While Google lets you a peek at places that once required a medical degree to access it does not make it easier to understand exactly what is going on with your health.

Customer service seems really high on the list of my job responsibilities these days. The thing is I don't really care about the surveys my bosses obsess over. I care about you. My focus has always been providing compassionate care with attention to details. Lucky for you, kindness mattered to me before it became a check box on a survey.

Also worth noting about me: I studied anatomy, physiology, nutrition, psychology, pharmacology, and gobs of nursing process to get here. My skills and knowledge have been tested. Getting those two letters RN was certainly no cake walk and regulations make me work hard to keep them.

Despite what you have 'heard' about nursing, I don't make 'bank' caring for you. I'd like you to know this is much more than just a paycheck for me. I am the doctor's eyes and ears, and honestly, the expert on you-while you are here. I dig that role and am proud to aid in your recovery.

I live by the golden rule, even under stressful circumstances I will continue. I'd like to ask you do the same. While I understand grumpiness because you feel bad I will not tolerate verbal abuse.

Now, since you're not an expert on this sick-stuff, a few words about what to expect here....I am going to invade your personal space. A lot. Sorry, it cannot be helped. I will do my best to preserve your dignity and privacy. Also, I know your shows are important to you but some things just have to get done before TV.

It is kind of noisy here and you will be woken up in the middle of a great nap more than once. I will control what I can for you. As much as it sucks, know up front that it will still be loud and you will not always be resting.

There will be a lot of information coming at you quickly. Stop me if + ask me to repeat if I go to fast. The last thing I want is for you to be unclear about your care because that creates fear; something we are trying to minimize. Ask me questions + remember no subject is taboo. You will not shock me.

The sign on your door that says NPO is a fancy way to say please do not eat anything. There is a reason for it. I know you are hungry but you will hate rescheduling your surgery+ paying for an extra day in care because 'Google said 4 hours was plenty of time to digest a cheeseburger'. It's going to be hard to endure the pain and vomiting you bring yourself if your tummies' not awake yet from that surgery. There is nothing at McDonalds worth the result of 'a small bite'; trust me on this one.

Call me before you get out of bed or before you decide to take a medication that you take at home but that the doctors have taken you off of at this time. Again, I ask for your trust to avoid unintended consequences for yourself.

I may be an expert on nursing stuff but I am not an expert on your body. If it feels weird, tell me, nothing is unimportant.

I promise to communicate clearly and directly with you. If you do the same, things will be as pleasant as possible for you. I will ask your understanding up front here. See, when you call for me to come help you I am usually helping your neighbor in the next bed. If I do not come running immediately when you call it does not mean that your pain is unimportant to me. It means I am giving outstanding care to a different patient. You have the right to know exactly what I am doing at all times. You have the right to help me plan your care. In fact, if possible I want you involved. You have the right to refuse care, too. You do not have the right to tell me how to nurse; regardless of how many nurses are in your family. I am a professional who would never come into your workplace and presume to know how you could perform better.

If you are expecting a Hilton-like experience you are going to be disappointed however; your needs will be met, I promise.

If you see me sitting at the desk, don't assume that means I have downtime. You would not believe the paperwork that you bring with you; every little thing you do must be documented. Lastly, you may see or hear me laughing from time-to-time. I hope you don't assume I am neglecting your care. Honestly, you never know what has just happened in the room next door. I may need that laugh to regroup myself, for both our benefit.

Most important, just in case you are wondering...I take you home with me each day. Your stay and your story help me count my own blessings and affirm what is important in my world. I examine the care I gave you microscopically and I treat you as I would my first born child. I pray as I leave each day that your body and the treatment will cooperate with one another so you get to go home and spend many more years with your loved ones and sometimes, when there is no more medicine, I ask that your death be peaceful and your family comforted as you leave them. Either way, I send up good thoughts for you from the moment that we meet. I hope that my care is so good that you do even remember my name the day after you leave here and I hope you know that you stay with me a long time after you are gone.

Your presence changed me and I am grateful for sharing this space with you; however brief. Let me thank you up front for that gift. It has been a blessing to care for you~Your Nurse

Author Afterward

Lastly, I need to thanks some folks:

- To that 'one' LVN in school that kept me company and reminded me I could trust
- To that 'one' professor who fought for our class and reminded me that some causes are worth the fight
- To that 'one' preceptor in school whose horrible actions ignited my passion to change the culture of nursing
- To that 'one' preceptor at my job that taught me how to hang in the ICU without losing my shit as a new nurse
- To that 'one' amazing new peer who lets me see she is overloaded, too
- To that 'one' man in my life who reminds me I am amazing
- To that 'one' friend who reminds me of my worth
- To that 'one' group of internet rebels who help me be my BOOM-tastic best
- To that 'one' shamanistic superhero who helped me find my superpower

You all continue to amaze me on a daily basis.

I will most likely never be able to thank you enough for your contributions to my life. I say thank you anyway....

I feel beyond blessed + honored to have shared some portion of my path with you all.

I appreciate everything you have done for me and all the ways you show me how 'one' person is all it takes to change the world. You will all have my gratitude forever.

Melissa Andersen is an RN, a wife, a mom, an
activist, artist, cyclist, life changer and badass.

She is on a mission to help the culture of nursing evolve by
showing each nurse how to locate their own unique medicine
and then how to share that medicine with the world.

Nursing is sacred work that needs some powerful magic.
Luckily each nurse carries within them a totally divine magic
that only that nurse can give to the world.

She does not plan on stopping until every single nurse
practices from that place of power within them.

She's creating this rEVOLution through private coaching,
group sessions, You Tube, podcasts, group talks, cycling and
all around merry-making.

Join her at www.nurseawesome.com

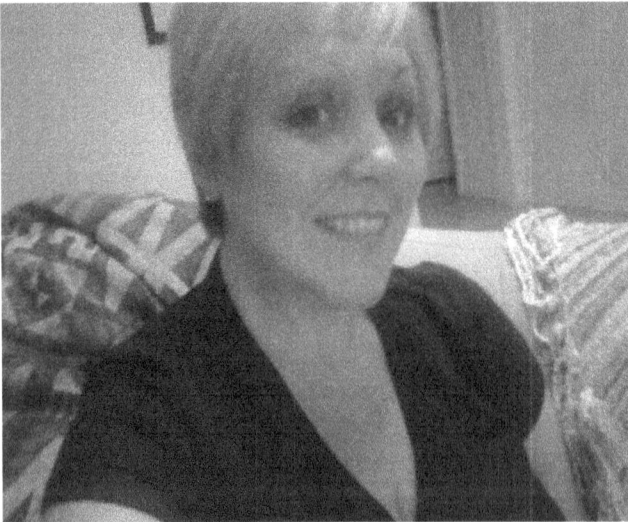

Disclaimer: While the events shared in this book are my experiences, there is a lot that has been changed. I know the HIPPA Gods watch everything and I have an awesome imagination so if you think anyone referenced here is a patient or person you know; you are wrong. Patient privacy is uber-important to me so the sexes and exact conditions of patients discussed in this book have been changed, twisted and combined with other stories in order to make a point and in order to protect the identity and privacy of the patient.